Lorenz

THE ARTIFICIAL INTELLIGENCE
REVOLUTION IN MEDICINE
How the forthcoming dermatology is shaping up

Index

"I would actually be very pessimistic about the World, if something like AI wasn't coming down the road."

Demis Hassabis, DeepMind co-founder, Economist
Innovation Summit, September 2018

"Everyone takes the limits of his own vision for the limits of the World."

Arthur Schopenhauer

Preamble

I would like to report in advance the reasons that led me to deal with a subject that can be considered atypical for a thesis of a medical student. I hope that the readers of my paper will appreciate its originality.

Everything begun a few years ago: since I was a child, I've always been interested in technology; at first, I was interested in computers and in the early rudimentary smartphones that, in those years, were beginning to be produced.
I used to spend my days reading magazines about phones and PCs and wondering how these technologies could have evolved in the future. I also used to draw bezel less smartphones with under-display cameras and fingerprints sensors, such as those that are currently on the market.

However, over the years, my attention has shifted from hardware to software.

In 2014 I bought some Facebook shares, and, from that lucky day on, I started to read daily news regarding the social-network giant and its board of directors.

I read articles about Mark Zuckerberg, David Marcus, Sharyl Sanderg, Yann LeCun, etc., as if I were reading the ones about my favorite football clubs and players.

Their attention for Artificial Intelligence brought me in contact for the first time with this new topic, so I started to scan everything I could find about it. Beginning with the basic considerations and premises, up to the strangest theories and scenarios.

All these themes, in the context of my thesis, will be gathered in the figure of the engineer, presented as a meeting point for all the quantitative subjects.

The figure of the engineer, in this paper, will be in contrast with that of the doctor, that will be representing the qualitative ones.

There will therefore be a dualism between what happens inside of the clinic and what happens outside of it.

This leads me to introduce the second character of my script, since, while reading these authors, I was attending Medical School, and I was very surprised by the fact that the issues that interested and interest me so much - AI on all - were never, or just briefly, addressed in class.

It is shocking, in fact; the whole World is talking about this technology: from the World leaders to the greatest engineers and entrepreneurs of our times, and everyone is competing to grab the limitless potential of this extraordinary invention; *how is it possible that we, as doctors, don't even talk about it?*

This is the exact point where my struggle begun, since I think that, out of the windows of our clinics, a revolution is taking place; a revolution that will upset our lives and that will affect the economic, ethical, medical and social spheres; however, inside of our clinics, we accept with suspicion these new technological discoveries and we take refuge in bygone praxis and in anachronistic habits, often covering our eyes in front of reality.

Why does it have to be this way?

Looking for an answer to this question, I searched for a figure that could connect the two apparently opposed worlds – the biomedical engineer, in the person of professor Cevenini.

I discovered that I could explore the convergence of these two scientific fields and I decided to deal with a thesis that deepened several aspects of artificial intelligence, involving present and future quantitative medicine.

Introduction

This thesis will address the issues related to the use of artificial intelligence in the medical field and, more specifically, in the dermatological field.

Although Medicine is not properly considered to be a quantitative science (Panda, 2006), but rather a semi-quantitative one, since ancient times, from the time of Hippocrates, in the fourth century BC, the Father of Medicine understood the importance of collecting and analyzing patient data (Mainland, 1952), as a representation of particular conditions that, until then, were simply considered with a qualitative descriptive approach.

However, we must wait until the seventeenth century for medicine to be considered a science, since when it began to follow the experimental scientific method of Galileo Galilei (Ascenzi, 1993).

It will be a colleague and a friend of Galilei himself, Santorio Santorio, the person that, in the same century, will carry out the first quantitative studies to evaluate the heart rate and that will also begin to make use of special machines, including specific thermometers, to support diagnosis and to the precisely objectivate definite clinical signs (Farina, 1975).

Santorio is also known to be the founder of **iatromechanics**, the science that considers the human organism as a set of various machinery – organs and apparatus – which can be educationally considered individually, and which can be represented through physical and mathematical models (Armocida, 1993).

Iatromechanics developed in the 17th century mainly thanks to both the English physician William Harvey, who first accurately described the cardiovascular system and hemodynamics (Aird, 2011), and the Italian anatomist-physiologist Marcello Malpighi, professor of theoretical medicine at the University of Bologna (Paolo Mandrioli, 2016).

Although, at the time, there was still a rudimentary knowledge of the functioning of apparatuses and organs, wanting to represent them faithfully through the physical and mathematical models to which they were traced, the use of increasingly refined technologies took on more and more ground, until reaching a central and cardinal role in clinical practice, up to the present day, in which imaging has an accuracy almost comparable to that of histology, and therefore superior to that of any semeiologist (Christopher Moriates, Krishan Soni, & Andrew Lai, 2013).

Over the centuries, however, it was realized that technological progress and the medical training necessary to adopt it evolved and improved at completely different rates (Thomas B. Sheridan, 2018).

This, which is one of the cornerstones of my thesis, has led to the creation of professional figures such as health technicians, first, and, later, of bio-engineers, able to put two apparently conflicting worlds, but that could enormously benefit one another, in communication: the Medical and the Engineering worlds (Mainland, 1952).

However, the still existing divergence was then accentuated by the introduction of computers, first, and artificial intelligences, then (Donald A. B. Lindberg & Betsy L. Humphreys, 1995).

In 1623, in fact, Willhelm Sickhart created a machine capable of performing mathematical calculations with numbers up to six digits; in the following year, Blaise Pascal built a machine able to do operations using the automatic carryover, while in 1674 Gottfried Wilhelm von Leibniz created a machine able to perform the sum, the difference and the multiplication in a recursive way (R.J. Anderson, 2018).

Between 1834 and 1837, Charles Babbage worked on the model of a machine called the analytical machine, whose characteristics partly anticipated those of modern computers (Hyman, 1982).

Another important step was the article by **Alan Turing** written in 1936, *"On Computable Numbers, With an Application to The*

Entscheidungsproblem", which lays the foundations for concepts such as calculability, computability, Turing machine, etc.: key definitions for computers up to the present day.

Later, in 1943, McCulloch and Pitts created what was considered the first work concerning artificial intelligence.
Their system employs a model of artificial neurons in which the state of such neurons can be "turned on" or "turned off," with a transition to "on" in the presence of stimuli caused by a sufficient number of surrounding neurons (Zhang & Zhang, Jul 1999).

Thus, McCulloch and Pitts came to show, for example, that any computable function can be represented by some network of neurons, and that all logical connectives can be implemented by a simple neural structure.

However, these new technologies, with unimaginable potential – to describe, replicate and even overcome the human mind – also carry many risks and, above all, in the medical field, are not always easy to adopt (Szolovits, 2019).

In the first chapter of the thesis, in fact, we will see how the artificial intelligences, outside of the clinical sphere, are already widely and daily adopted: just think of the voice assistants, the algorithms of social networks, the email filters, the fact that sites and apps show us more and more customized content, or even content made specifically for us.

But these technologies have found a way to express their potential even in the physical world, with, for example, electric cars, robots, and the automation of increasingly complex tasks, leading also to potential problems such as, the more foregone, unemployment (Anton Korinek, December 2017).

In the medical world, on the other hand, the relationship between doctors and technologies is often troubled, as it will be described in the third chapter of the script, and, to better understand the potential benefits, risks and troubles of AIM, Artificial Intelligence in Medicine, the application of the iDScore model in Siena Dermatology Department will be taken as an example (L. Tognetti, 2018).

Even in the medical field, in fact, we are beginning to understand the enormous benefit that a doctor could derive from diagnostic support systems based on artificial intelligences, therefore allowing himself to be supported by the figure of the engineer (Informa Markets, 2019).

Many tech companies, including companies that have little to do with medicine, in fact, are focusing their efforts on the development of similar models and, through conferences and international fairs, such as Medica, the medical world is slowly beginning to become aware of the new technologies (Topol, 2019).

This will lead to the presentation of future perspectives that may have such important implications (the increase in diagnostic accuracy, the reduction of its costs and times, etc.) as risky ones: technologies able to replicate and overcome the human mind, in fact, if at first it is probable that they will just lead to manageable problems such as unemployment, in more distant future may even put Humanity in front of existential risk (Karan Narain, May 2019).

The scientific community, in the figure of the doctor, can no longer hide from these responsibilities nor continue to adapt so slowly to change.

"When I go around in my everyday life, I play the game "Find the Robot".
I go to the supermarket and I don't see any.
I go to the restaurant and I don't see robots.
I do not see them in the hospital, nor in the company I work for,
and, ultimately, I think we are very far from robotization."
Robert James Gordon, American economist, 5 June 2018,
Brussels Economic Forum

Chapter 1.

Artificial intelligence in the world

1.1 – Meaning of artificial intelligence

The first chapter of my paper will focus on the infinite applications that artificial intelligences are finding outside of the medical world.

The chapter aims to underline how these technologies, although perceived in clinical practice as abstract and distant, are in fact already heavily reshaping society and, above all, are being used practically by everyone every day, without even realizing it.

Therefore, experts are discussing how these technologies will reshape society.

Debate that, in the medical world, is guilty avoided.

To a brief introduction to AI, its main applications presentation will follow, and, in the last section of the chapter, the added value and the future perspectives of the use of Artificial Intelligence will be discussed.

In computer science, Artificial Intelligence (AI), is intelligence demonstrated by machines, in contrast to the natural intelligence, the one that is displayed by human beings.

Colloquially, the term is often associated with cognitive functions that we tend to associate with the natural intelligence of human mind, such as problem solving and learning.

As AIs become increasingly capable of solving always more complex problems, these tasks are often removed from the definition of AI; this phenomenon is known as the **AI effect**.

"AI is whatever hasn't been done yet."
Tesler's Theorem

This is enough to show how this issue is on the border between science and philosophy.

AI can be classified into three different types of systems:

- *Analytical*, that consists in cognitive intelligence, a long-debated philosophical conception based on the capability of the human mind to represent the environment. In the next chapters I will show how this is one of the greatest problems not only in the definition of AI, but also in the definition of Intelligence itself. The issue can be summarized by **The Problem of Other Minds**: *"Given that I can only observe the behavior of others, how can I know that others have minds?"*.

- *Human-inspired*, based both on cognitive and emotional intelligence, it's the capability to understand not only the environment, but also human emotions, taking them in consideration in the decision-making process.

- *Humanized artificial intelligence*, instead, summarizes all types of human competences, being the ability to be both self-conscious and self-aware in the interaction with other beings.

In the medical field, starting with analytical Artificial Intelligence, the most basic of these systems, often used in epidemiological research and for patients and resource management, we are starting to adopt human inspired and humanized AI, in order to interact directly with the patient, such as trough robotic nurses or chat bots that can provide psychological support or psychiatric advices.

However, there are still differences between natural and artificial intelligence.

AI algorithms, in fact, are dissimilar from human beings, in two ways:

1. Algorithms are *literal*: once a goal is set, there is no way to change it during the elaboration of the data.
   This means that, not only humans need to pay close attention to the goal that they are setting, but also that these algorithms need a lot of testing, in order to be sure that they are completing their task in the way that we wanted them to.

2. All algorithms are *black boxes*. This means that they can perfectly complete their task in the way that they are told to, but they are not yet able to give us an explanation on how they got to that result.

An example could be the one of an AI that, given the medical records of some patients and asked to predict the clinical history of other patients just by reading the first part of their medical records, correctly predicted the ones that were going to suffer from schizophrenia (Sunil Vasu Kalmady, 2019).

What was the problem, then?

Not only none taught to the AI how to predict schizophrenic trait, but trained psychiatrists are not able to do it themselves, since schizophrenia is an obscure illness whose exact pathogenesis is still not known.

How can we know how the AI at issue performed a task that not even its programmers know how to accomplish?

The answer is simple: we can't – yet.

What will it lead us to? What will it happen when artificial intelligence will become better than humans in doing their jobs? Will they leave all of us unemployed?

The greatest minds of our times are trying to give an answer to these questions.

On June 2018, in fact, at Brussels Economic Forum, two of the greatest World experts of Artificial Intelligence's economics debated on whether AI and automation were going to create or disrupt jobs.

On one side there was **Robert James Gordon**, American economist and Stanley G. Harris Professor of the Social Sciences at Northwestern University; on the other, **Jeremy Rifkin**, American economic and social theorist, writer, public speaker, political advisor, and activist.

Rifkin supported the thesis claiming that artificial intelligences would become so advanced as to destroy almost all the jobs, while Gordon claimed that every new technology, despite initial fears, creates way more jobs than it actually destroys.

The canonical example is that of the plow in farming: even though it took away a man's job; by increasing the production of goods and decreasing its costs, it gave to the economy the boost it needed to create more well-being and therefore new workplaces.
The same can be said for all the new technologies: from tools and machinery, to computers and Artificial Intelligence.

Gordon's position is based on three main assumptions:

- The jobs are not a finite datum, neither in the typology, nor in the number.

Every product, every market, every new technology, also creates new jobs: when one job dies, if the market works, another one, or even more than one, are created.

- A new work-technology replacement, in order to be adopted, must be cost-effective. This means that the existence of substitute labor technologies does not necessarily mean that those technologies will be adopted by companies.

- Technology evolves, but it is far from being able to replace complex jobs, which will remain exclusively human for a long time.

R. Gordon concludes his argument with the provocative phrase quoted at the beginning of the chapter, and that is the main point of his thesis, by simply saying that he doesn't see any robot.

Who is right, then?

In order to answer to this question, ZipRecruiter's data scientists analyzed over 50 million job postings, charted hundreds of employers, and thousands of job seekers, and examined specific use cases in five transitioning industries.

The result of their study was that AI created about three times as many jobs as it took away in 2018.

What's more, while employers are already using AI tools, 81% of those surveyed said they preferred to hire a human over putting in a completely autonomous system (ZipRecruiter, 2019).

The study also shows precisely the jobs that AI has created:

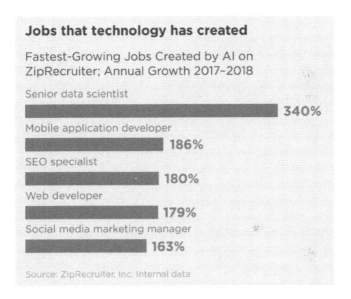

As shown in the graphic: senior data scientist, mobile application developer and SEO specialist are the three main jobs created by technology in 2018.

AI also creates new jobs directly by the need of experts that its development requires:

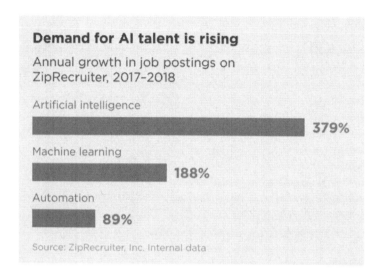

In just a year, the demand for jobs related to AI has risen by 379%.

For now, a similar consideration can be done also for the medical field, as shown in the following figure:

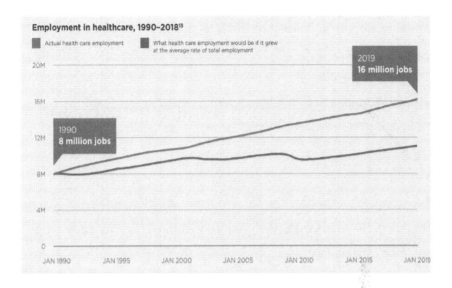

Employment in healthcare, 1990–2018[13]

- Actual health care employment
- What health care employment would be if it grew at the average rate of total employment

The graph shows that the employment rate in healthcare has risen faster than the average of total employment from January 1990 to January 2019, also thanks to the adoption of Artificial Intelligence in medical practice. However, this topic will be largely discussed in the next chapters.

Also, in California, where the **Silicon Valley** is located, unemployment rate fell to record-low 4.4% in 2018, gaining 35500 jobs (Khouri, March 2018).

In the U.K., instead, automation has created 3.5 million high-skilled jobs over the past 15 years, according to a 2017 workforce study by Deloitte, a consultancy firm.

Industrial employment in Germany is expected to rise by 1.8% by 2021, according to the Germany-based Center for European Economic Research.

Also, in Asia, as told by the Asian Development Bank in April 2018, automation has created an extra 34 million jobs (Yang, July 2019).

The question seems to be answered, then: as in every technological revolution, the new technology creates new jobs, therefore, the workforce is not wasted, but just redistributed; the same considerations can also be applied to the introduction of artificial intelligences – it seems.

However, Gordon's third and most important assumption needs to be re-analyzed.

The condition for jobs to be created and not disrupted, was that the technology didn't surpass human workforce in a specific task and that it didn't acquire the ability to perform complex jobs.

As we will see in detail in the next section of the chapter, this condition is not always satisfied.

It is logical to think that, in the future, artificial intelligence will surpass or at least equal natural one. But when will it happen?

Before answering to this question, we must describe the current condition of artificial intelligence-related jobs and think about the rate at which its evolution is occurring.

There are many fields in which AI complexity has gained an incredibly high degree, such as Atari games, chess, Go, shogi (Japanese chess) and, in the last days, also poker (Silver et al., 2017).

The board game **Go** deserves a separate reflection, in order to better understand the level at which AIs work.

Lee Sedol, 18-time world champion professional Go player, was defeated by **DeepMind**'s computer program AlphaGo in a 1–4 series in March 2016, the match has also been compared with the historic chess match between Deep Blue and Garry Kasparov in 1997, but this is only the premise.

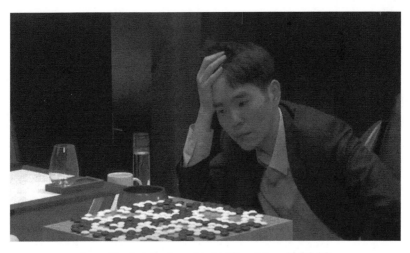

Lee Sedol facing AlphaGo, March 2016

On 19 October 2017, in fact, AlphaGo's team published an article on the journal Nature introducing AlphaGo Zero, a version created without using data from human games, and stronger than any previous version (Silver et al., 2017)

By playing games against itself, AlphaGo Zero surpassed the strength of AlphaGo Lee in *three days* by winning *100 games to 0*, reached the level of AlphaGo Master in 21 days, and exceeded all the old versions in 40 days (Hassabis, 2017).

Demis Hassabis, DeepMind co-founder and CEO, stated that AlphaGo Zero was so powerful because it was "no longer constrained by the limits of human knowledge" (Knapton, 2017).

AlphaGo Zero performances posed a new and great problem: if it was easy to estimate AlphaGo's intelligence/problem solving power, since it defeated a World champion 1-4, the same couldn't be said about AlphaGo Zero's, since its performances are at a level that *human mind can't even conceive.*

What if this superhuman intelligence is exported also to other fields? And, above all: how long will it take to do so?

In order to answer to these questions, let's start from the description of the current state of the art, and from the jobs that it is easier to automate in the coming years.

Within the coming years, in fact, sectors as agriculture and farming, finance, journalism, customer service, surveillance, retail, driving, delivery and law are going to be heavily influenced by the introduction of artificial intelligence.

AI poses a real and enormous threat to the work force of this fields and, moreover, to the structure of our society.

As time passes, a crescent number of jobs will be lost to automation and a crescent number of people will be left unemployed.

On the long run, how are the governments going to handle the increasingly high unemployment rate?

Another important consideration about this topic concerns the speed with which they are improved, adopted and used.

A very huge mistake comes from the belief that the speed with which these technologies improve follows a linear course, instead, this trend is exponential, as Raymond Kurzweil, one of the pioneers and the world's greatest experts in this field, says.

Raymond Kurzweil (New York, February 12, 1948), Google Director of Engineering, is an American inventor and futurist, that in 1999 wrote a book – *"The Age of Spiritual Machines"* – in which he introduced the *The Law of Accelerating Returns*, further explained in a 2001 essay named after his revolutionary theory.

To explain it with his words:

"An analysis of the history of technology shows that technological change is exponential, contrary to the common-sense 'intuitive linear' view. So, we won't experience 100 years of progress in the 21st century—it will be more like 20,000 years of progress (at today's rate). The 'returns,' such as chip speed and cost-effectiveness, also increase exponentially. There's even exponential growth in the rate of exponential growth. Within a few decades, machine intelligence will surpass human intelligence, leading to the Singularity—technological change so rapid and profound it represents a rupture in the fabric of human history. The implications include the merger of biological and nonbiological intelligence, immortal software-based humans, and ultra-high levels of intelligence that expand outward in the universe at the speed of light."

His assumptions largely are based on *Moore's Law* (1965): described as the observation that the number of transistors in a dense integrated circuit doubles about every two years (Moore, April 19, 1965).
Gordon Earle Moore (born January 3, 1929) is the co-founder and chairman emeritus of **Intel Corporation**.

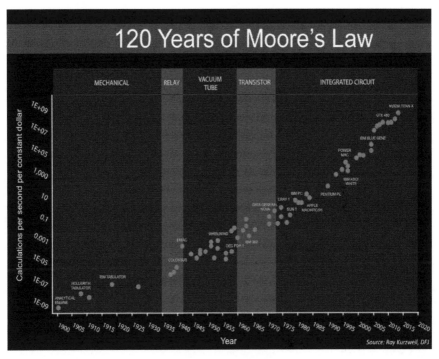

(By Steve Jurvetson)

Kurweil's graph shows, as an example, the application of Moore's Law to the calculation per second per constant dollar performed by a processor.

Sounds crazy, right? And it would be, were it not for the fact that the World's leading tech entrepreneurs share the same theories and fears exposed by Ray Kurzweil.

In fact, Elon Musk has founded the company **Neuralink** in order to combine artificial intelligence with natural intelligence, thus making the latter immortal, and shares Kurzweil's worries also with Masayoshi Son, CEO of **SoftBank** and founder of the $100 billion Vision fund, Jack Ma, 21st richest men of the World and executive chair of **Alibaba Group**, Mark Zuckerberg, CEO of **Facebook**, which however has a more racy vision, Bill Gates, CEO of **Microsoft**, and, until last year, with the famous theoretical physicist Stephen Hawking, as well as many others.

Many theories, that will be presented in the last sections of this script, are rising, spacing from Universal Basic Income, UBI, that is already being tested around the Globe, to Fully Automated Luxury Communism.

These issues, of absolute and transversal importance, as said, will be taken up in the last chapter of the script.

For now, what is important is to emphasize how the whole world is taking an interest in these technologies, adopting them, and discussing their implications and consequences on a daily basis.

Although the medical world is completely foreign to these arguments, World leaders, scientists, entrepreneurs and engineers debate these themes every day.

The following are the fields in which the technological revolution is already taking place.

1.2 – Main applications

Farming

"I think agriculture is the greatest near-term — I define over the next five years — opportunity around robotics and autonomy."
		Loup Ventures managing partner Gene Munster (Larkin, October 2018)

Farming is one of the eldest and most central professions in the world. Worldwide, agriculture is a $5 trillion industry, and now the industry is turning to AI technologies to yield healthier crops, control pests, monitor growing conditions and soil, organize data, help with workload, and improve a wide variety of tasks in the entire food supply chain.

AI systems are also helping to progress harvest quality – what is known as **precision agriculture**.

Precision agriculture makes use of AI technology to aid in detecting diseases in plants, pests, and poor plant nutrition.

Forecasts say that, by 2020, farmers will be using 75 million connected devices. Moreover, by 2050, an average farm is expected to generate an average of 4.1 million data points every day (Forbes, 2019).

Farming is also facing the big problem of workers shortage: one solution to help with this problem is AI agriculture bots.

These bots enlarge the human labor personnel and are used in numerous forms. The bots can harvest crops at a higher volume and faster pace than human employees, more accurately identify and eradicate weeds, and lesser costs for farms by having around the clock labor force.

Other possible examples of AI driven agriculture include, among the others, drones, driverless tractors, automated irrigation systems and facial recognition of domestic cattle (Forbes, 2019).

In 2018, Iron Ox opened its first automated farm (Vincent, October 2018) and, by the end of the year, Driscoll, one of America's largest berry producer and distributor, will be fielding its harvesters with its robot farmers (Larkin, October 2018).

This explains the sentence written at the beginning of the paragraph and underlines how the adoption of new technologies in farming is much closer and faster than in many other fields.

Journalism

"Maybe a few years ago A.I. was this new shiny technology used by high tech companies, but now it's actually becoming a necessity."
Francesco Marconi, head of research and development at The Journal (NYT, 2019).

As journalists and editors often find themselves the victims of layoffs at digital publishers and traditional newspaper chains, machine generated journalism is on the rise.

For instance, roughly a third of the content published by Bloomberg News uses some form of Artificial Intelligence. The system used by the company, **Cyborg**, is able to assist reporters in churning out thousands of articles on company earnings reports each quarter.

The algorithms can dissect a financial report the exact moment it appears and spit out an immediate news story that includes the most pertinent facts and figures. This work is done 24 hours a day 7 days a week, without typos, pauses, and complaints.

Also, The Guardian's Australia, Forbes, The Post, The Wall Street Journal, Dow Jones, and many other news companies use similar technologies (Peiser, 2019).

In 2018, China also presented the World first news anchor that will report tirelessly all day every day, from everywhere in the country (Kuo, November 2018).

"I, who was wholly cloned from a real-life host, have mastered broadcasting as well as the real host.
As long as I am provided with text, I can speak as a news host."
AI anchor (Kuo, November 2018).

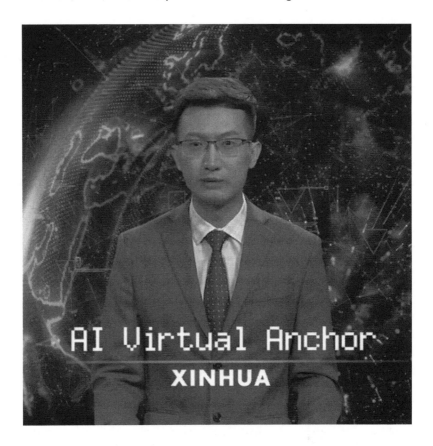

In the same year, 2018, Artificial Intelligence has also been able to write novels (Hornigold, Oct 25, 2018) and, in the following year, textbooks (Vincent, April 2019).

The next section will try to answer to the questions that editors are asking themseves: how long will it take to AI to get rid of human jurnalists and anchors?

Driving

Elon Musk (June 28, 1971), 25th most powerful man on the Planet (Forbes, 2019) and 40th-richest person in the World (Forbes, 2019), is a technology entrepreneur, investor, and engineer.

He is the co-founder of PayPal (2000), founder, CEO, and lead designer of SpaceX (2002), co-founder, CEO, and product architect of **Tesla, Inc.** (2003), co-founder and co-chairman of OpenAI (2015), co-founder and CEO of Neuralink (2016), and founder of The Boring Company (2016).

Many of the companies that he founded are related to the topic of my thesis, however, this section of my script will only focus on Tesla and, more generally, on autonomous cars.

On July 17, Tesla stated that it is ready to commercialize fully self-driving cars as soon as this year, and that this is going to be done through an over-the-air update to hundreds of thousands of cars, and, because of the fact that autonomous vehicles are largely self-regulated — guided by industries but with no clearly enforceable rules — no one can stop the automaker from moving ahead.

The statement rose a large amount of criticism and perplexities, but Tesla seems not worried about it, since, as it claims, its AI's have been collecting data from all their cars all over the World since the first one of them hit the road (Siddiqui, July 17, 2019).

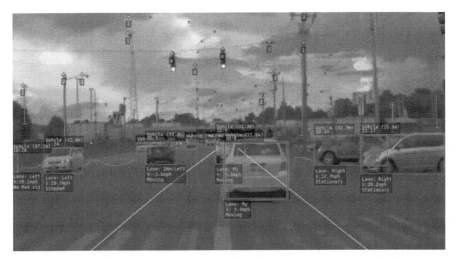

Tesla's AI-based driving system (tesla.com)

Nevertheless, a lot of other companies, such as Waymo, General Motors, Nissan, Delphi Automotive Systems, Bosch, Mercedes Benz, BMW, Ford, Volkswagen and many others, are actively testing this technology (Wang, 2018).

How long will it take to this companies to take over jobs such as taxi, bus and camion driver, just to cite a few?
Above all, is the World ready to welcome this imminent change?

43

Retail

"Amazon Go is a new kind of store featuring the world's most advanced shopping technology. No lines, no checkout – just grab and go!"
Amazon.com

Amazon Go is a chain of convenience stores in the U.S. operated by Amazon, with four locations, each in Chicago and Seattle, two in San Francisco, and one in New York as of May 2019 (Amazon.com).

Customers are able to buy products without being checked out by a human cashier or using a self-checkout station: through AI, customers and their purchases are tracked within the store, making human cashiers useless.

In the early stages, Amazon Go stores were also cash-less, but this was considered discriminatory for low-income customers, and forced Amazon to accept also cash payments (Har, May 7, 2019).

In September 2018, Bloomberg reported that Amazon was considering opening 3000 Amazon Go locations across the United States by 2021.

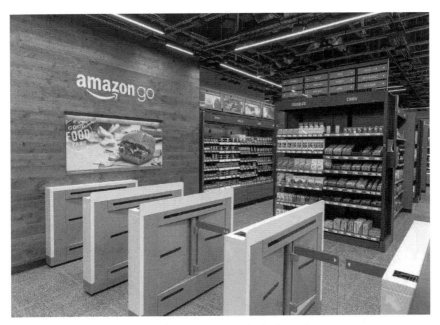

One of Amazon Go's locations.

Jeff Bezos' company, however, is not the only one that's betting big on automated retail: JD, Alibaba (China's Amazon), Walmart, Kroger, Jack&Jones, Hema, Lotte and many others are gearing up in order to raise against Amazon's predominance (Nick Wingfield, 2018).

In this case, beyond the problem of possible unemployment that can result from the introduction of these technologies, as we will

45

see also in the next chapter, the greatest concern of customers regards the processing of their **personal data**.

Is it right for Amazon to have all this information on our behavior?

Data on what we eat, how much we drink, where we are, how much we spend, even in the real-life offline world, will be saved in their servers and repeatedly analyzed by their algorithms – *forever*.

As we will see in the section of this chapter on surveillance, in the eyes of many, the aforementioned technologies introduce a perspective that confronts us with a possible establishment of an **Orwellian regime**, leading us to ask ourselves if this is what we really want.

Customer Service and Contact Centre

"Customers can ask the Google Assistant to make phone calls on their behalf, for tasks like booking an appointment or checking your business hours. The Assistant will confirm any necessary details with the customer and call your business to fulfill the customer's request."

(Google.com)

In May 2018, on the stage of I/O, the 47 years old **Sundar Pichai**, Google CEO, showed off a jaw-dropping new capability of Google Assistant: the ability to make phone calls on the behalf of customers (Welch, 2018).

Google Assistant, released in May 2016, is an AI powered virtual assistant developed by Google available on smartphones and smart home devices, falling therefore in the vast categories of Internet of Things (Iot) and Industry 4.0, and installed on more than 400 million devices in 2017 (Rijo, 2017).

Beyond the extraordinary performance of the voice assistant, what is stanning, is the possibility of technologies like this to replace millions of phone operators, phone assistants and secretaries.

In fact, according to Gartner Projections, up to 85% of customer interactions will be managed without human involvement by 2020 (Frazzetto, 2018) and, according to Gartner analyst Brian Manusama, "countries like India may have a huge problem with increasing unemployment" (Baraniuk, 2018).

At this point, it could be argued that, as true as it is that Artificial Intelligence has led us to the gates of a social revolution, what it is still limited to is automating low-labor jobs, currently carried out mainly by poorly educated people.

The level of complexity of the jobs described in the next examples will therefore be a little higher.

Trading

"Artificial intelligence is to trading what fire was to the cavemen."
(Thomas, 2019).

In 2016, the Hong Kong based company **Aidiya** got renowned because it started a hedge fund that completed all operational transaction through AI solely, without any involvement of humans. The founder of Aidiya is famous for the following quote about his company: *"If we all die, it'll still continue to trade"* (Zamagna, 2018).

According to a recent study by U.K. research firm Coalition, artificial trades account for almost 45% of revenues in cash equities trading, this shouldn't be surprising, since, already in

2017, as JPMorgan reported, traditional traders represented a mere 10% of trading volume (Thomas, 2019).

Some of the tasks in which artificial intelligence is already being used include:

- Sentiment analysis,
- Forecast and predictions,
- Blockchain analysis,
- Fundamental analysis,
   (Zamagna, 2018).

Also, **Morgan Stanley** used AI to study its own analysts' performances and this approach showed a solid performance between January 2013 and May 2019 period, with a positive return in 2018 versus the market's 5% drop (Franck, June 2019).

These are just some examples of how AI has already reached superhuman performances and is already being widely used in this sector.

What will it lead us to? *"In 10 years, Goldman Sachs will be significantly smaller by head count than it is today"*, Daniel Nadler, CEO of Kensho, told The New York Times, and, about the people left unemployed, Minevich, author and world-renowned visionary in the fields of digitization and AI, added on the topic: "Some of these smart people will move into tech startups, or will help develop more AI platforms, or autonomous cars, or energy technology" (SciPol, 2019)

A fair exchange, isn't it? AI works for us and we work for it, as seen in the previous section of this chapter.

Legal Practice

"What is the law but a series of algorithms?"
(Sahota, Forbes, 2019).

To the day, in legal framework, AI is being used to conduct time-consuming research, reducing the burdens on courts and legal services and quickening the judicial procedure.

There are also situations where using AI might be preferable to interacting with a human, such as for client interviews. For instance, it's been demonstrated that people are more likely to be honest with a machine than with a person, since a machine isn't capable of judgment – yet (Sahota, Forbes, 2019).

The following are the main tasks that AI is already taking on:

- Review documents and legal research
- Help perform due diligence
- Contract review and management
- Predict legal outcomes
- Automating divorce
  (Marr, 2018)

Also, as soon as in 2018, 20 top lawyers were brutally defeated by a legal AI - LawGeex AI software's accuracy was accounted for 94% in 26 seconds, compared to an average of 85% for lawyers with an average time of 92 minutes - (Bechor, 2018) and, in the same year, Deloitte forecasted that 100000 legal roles will be automated by 2036.

The legal company reported that, by 2020, law firms will be faced with a "tipping point" for a new talent strategy and that NextLaw Labs was also planning to found "the first legal technology venture created by a law firm".

It is not a case that PricewaterhouseCoopers named 2020 the **"Decade of Disruption"** – and it is only 2 months apart from my degree discussion.

The following and last example of this section is perhaps the most significative: although it does not cause many job losses, compared to the other possible AI employments presented in this chapter, it epitomizes the application of artificial intelligence from which the greatest repercussions on society can arise in the near term, and its introduction is therefore often accompanied by harsh criticism and firm opposition from many people all over the World.

Surveillance

"...always eyes watching you and the voice enveloping you. Asleep or awake, indoors or out of doors, in the bath or bed—no escape. Nothing was your own except the few cubic centimeters in your skull."
George Orwell, "1984".

The **Social Credit System**, SCC, is a national reputation system that is being developed by the Chinese Government, that, by 2020, plans to standardize the social reputation of its citizens and businesses.

The system is based mostly on image recognition and big data, both fueled by Artificial Intelligence, as we will see in detail in the second chapter of the script.

Last year, in 2018, some restrictions have already been placed on citizens and this has been seen as one of the first steps toward the institution of the Nationwide SCC.

The Government's plan is to **rank citizens** based on their social credit and to reward or punish them accordingly.

Everything a citizen does is taken into account: buying diapers or paying bills on time can rise their score; buying alcohol or even non-essential items, instead, can lower it, as well as cheating in videogames, playing them for many hours in a single day, spreading fake news, refusing military service, watching porn or visiting unreliable websites.

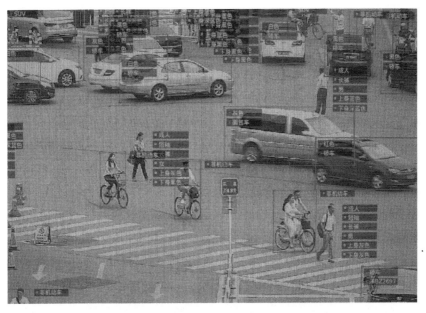

How China's SCC works (Bloomberg)

Every citizen starts off with a score of 1000 points, that can be lost through incorrect behavior, creating a ranking and various citizen classes.

NPR reported the ranking as follows:

- 960 to 1000 is an A;
- 850 to 955 points is a B;
- 840 to 600 is a C;
- Any score below that is a D, which means the score-holder is "untrustworthy."

"Bad" citizens are then disciplined by the System, and the punishments include:

- Banning them from flying or getting the train - the system has been used to already block 9 million people with "low scores" from purchasing domestic flights,
- Throttling their internet speeds,
- Banning them — or their kids — from the best schools,
- Stopping them from getting the best jobs,
- Keeping them out of the best hotels,

- Getting their dog/s taken away,
- Being publicly named as bad citizens,

The good citizens, instead, are rewarded by getting more matches on dating websites and discounts on energy bills, renting things without deposits and getting better interest rates at banks (Ma, 2018).

Disputes concerning the System are as obvious as numerous and will be presented in the third chapter of this paper.
What can be asked, for now, is how close we are to this future, and, now that we have a wider view, how it can impact public health.

What would happen if governments collected all the available data concerning a person's health? Not only the medical records, but also how many cigarettes, alcohol, vegetables or sweets a person consumes, if he goes to run, is registered in the gym, buys the medicines that is prescribed and what would happen if the State could reward him or punish him according to his behavior.

The next section will be centered on the advantages that AI can bring to the social sphere outside of Medicine; in the next chapter, instead, we will talk about how the same technologies are impacting medical practice.

1.3 - Added value and future perspective

As presented in the previous section, and according to **Forbes Technology Council**, an invitation-only community for world-class CIOs, CTOs and technology executives, the most important ways in which Artificial Intelligence can benefit society, instead of harming it, are the following:

- Enhancement of efficiency and throughput, since machines are able to work tirelessly 24 hours a day and 7 days a week, without pauses and decline in concentration.

- Increasement of automation: as mentioned, all repetitive low-labor jobs will be automated within a few years. Then it will be the turn of the more complex ones.

- Benefit for multiple industries: in addition to those mentioned, there are many other industries that can be automated - catering, cooking, home deliveries, cleaning, education, etc.

- Adding Jobs and strengthening the economy, as shown by professor Gordon in the first part of this chapter,

- Massive reduction of errors: this is an important point for my thesis and will be further developed in the following sections.
  In addition to tirelessness, an important merit of AI is the fact that it can't commit errors, unless it's taught to.

- Permitting next generation disaster response, as an example of situation in which specific protocols must be followed, and it must be done quickly, without hesitations and errors.

- Solution of complex social problems: beyond criticism, that will be discussed in the following chapters, the use of AI in surveillance can guarantee a safer and healthier society.

- Leading to loss of control: paradoxically, technologies such as AI can be applied in order to create impartial judges, incorruptible policemen and super partes legislators, giving up the control of the system to more balanced and fairer intelligences than the natural one.

- Absolution of humans of many responsibilities: as in the previous point, by giving up to some of its power, mankind can also give up on many to its responsibilities.

- Enhancement of Human lifestyle: Human lifestyle will also benefit from the massive automation of repetitive tasks that the new technologies are already introducing. Google Assistant, as well as IoT, were just some early examples of how AI can make Human life a lot easier.

- Elevation of the condition of Mankind: fewer working hours, a better lifestyle in a healthier and safer environment, in a more equal and decentralized social system, can eventually uplift Human condition.

- Freeing up of Humans to do what they do best: many people are spending their entire lives doing a low-labor job that doesn't fit their liking nor their qualities. AI has the power to change this condition - whether for better or for worse is yet to be seen.

- Extension and expansion of creativity: liberated from repetitive tasks and from many working hours, Humans could eventually do what's traditionally considered to differentiate them from machines.

(Forbes Technology Council, 2018).

Speaking of **future perspectives**, according to a 2019 study from Oxford Economics, robots could take over 20 million manufacturing jobs around the World by 2030, and, within the next 11 years, there could be 14 million robots put to work in China alone.

Moreover, if robot installations were boosted to 30% more than the baseline forecast by 2030, researchers estimated it would lead to a 5.3% boost in global GDP that year: "This equates to adding an extra $4.9 trillion per year to the global economy by 2030 - equivalent to an economy greater than the projected size of Germany's", the report said (Taylor, June 2019).

All roses, then? Yes – at least for this chapter.

The central point of this section is to present the main strengths of AI and advantages that this new technology can bring to mankind.

These benefits are not ideal or imaginary, but, as shown in the previous section, they are real, current and substantial.

How does the medical world relate to these new technologies? Is their adoption as quick and efficient as it has been in many, if not all, of the other fields?

"The Caterpillar-on-the-Leaf Syndrome.
A typical defect of all specialized professions is that, by
continuing to study the leaf, one ends up thinking that its ribs are
the only thing that exist in the World."
Dr. N. Nante, Hygiene and Public Health professor, University of
Siena

Chapter 2.

Artificial intelligence in Medicine

2.1– The current state of AI in the medical field

In contrast to the previous one, this chapter will focus on the use of artificial intelligences in the medical field.

In the first section of the chapter, a brief introduction to the history of AI in medical practice will be followed by the presentation of the current state of its adoption.

The second section, instead, will present some examples of this new technology in the clinic.

I would like that, while reading this chapter, the doctors began to feel called into question and asked themselves, example after example, if they had ever seen or used the technologies presented.

The history of Artificial Intelligence in Medicine, AIM, begins in the **1960s**, with Dendral, a problem-solving program, also known as *expert system*.

Dendral, acronym of the term "Dendritic Algorithm", was created at Stanford University by E. Feigenbaum, B. G. Buchanan, J. Lederberg, and C. Djerassi, along with a team of research associates and students.

This project began in 1965 and spans approximately half the history of AI research. His aim was to help organic chemists in identifying unknown organic molecules, by analyzing their mass spectra and using the knowledge of chemistry of that time.

It was the first program to be considered an expert system because it automated the decision-making process of chemists.

Organization of the heuristic DENDRAL programs

Operation	Components	Input	Output
Planning	MOLION	Mass spectrum	Molecular ion constraints
	Planning rule generator	Planning rules	Constraints
	PLANNER	Planning rules	Superatoms GOODLIST BADLIST
Generating	Acyclic generator CONGEN GENOA STEREO	Constraints	Candidate molecular structures
Testing	PREDICTOR	Candidate molecular structures	Most plausible structures
	MSPRUNE	Mass spectrometry rules	Structures consistent with spectrum
	REACT	Reaction chemistry rules	Structures consistent with known reactions

A table from Dendral (Semantic Scholar)

Dendral was written in LISP programming language, the second-oldest high-level programming language in widespread use today, designed by John McCarthy – the father of the term "Artificial Intelligence".

Even though it was written for chemistry, it provided the bases for one of the most significant early uses of AI in Medicine: MYCIN, as well as other systems, such as INTERNIST-1 and CASNET.

MYCIN, whose name derives from the suffix of macrolide antibiotics, "-mycin", was a backward chaining expert system that used AI to identify bacteria causing severe infections (e.g.:

meningitis) and to recommend antibiotics, with the dosage adjusted for patient's weight.

It has been developed in the early **1970s** at Stanford University and it was written in LISP, as well as Dendral.

In its results, MYCIN received an acceptability rating of 65% on treatment plan from eight independent specialists, which was comparable to the 42.5% to 62.5% rating of five faculty members.

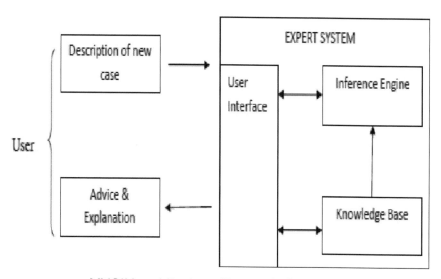

MYCIN architecture (Semantic Scholar)

Given its outstanding performance, we could expect it to be adopted by all the doctors of the developed World. But it didn't go as expected; in fact, *Mycin was never used in clinical practice.*

But why? At that time, the state of technologies for the system integration wasn't ready to run this program. Nonetheless, numerous legal and ethical issues around the use of computers in medical practice were raised.

Therefore, in the 70s, with the birth of the first AIM, an important reflection also raised: *should we use it?* If not, why?

Even INTERNIST-1, designed to reproduce the behavior of a diagnostician, and CASNET, a consultant to ophthalmologists for complex cases of glaucoma, met the same fate, not achieving routine use by practitioners.

1980s and **1990s** have been marked by the following themes, that led to a wider spread of AI within the hospitals:

- Emergence of HIS, Hospital Information System, focused on the administrational needs of hospitals,
- Financial information, easily quantifiable, was taken into account as well as clinical information,
- Introduction of PC's into offices brought thousands of doctors in contact with technology, first, and AI, after,
- PCs were also integrated to units for data output,

- Health Level Seven International (HL7) foundation, an organization dedicated to providing standards and solutions that empower global health data interoperability.

During this time, there was a recognition by researchers and developers that AI systems in healthcare must be designed to accommodate these two conditions:

- The absence of perfect data. Being considered a semi-quantitative subject, Medicine can't be perfectly represented by mathematical models
- AIs should be built on the knowledge of physicians. (Miller, 1994)

In the early **2000s,** the technological advancements that have enabled the growth of healthcare-related applications of AI included:

- The exponential growth of computer power and the consequenting decrease of its costs have enabled faster and wider data collection and processing,
- The increased amount of data acquired through health-related devices and wearables led to an enormous amount of information,

- The growth of genomic sequencing databases, topic that interests me personally, being an *Illumina* shareholder,
- The advancements in natural language processing and computer vision, allowing machines to imitate human perceptual processes,
- The improved accuracy of robot-assisted surgery.

This leads us to the **modern days** and where we can find the application of AIM.

Medical practice, in dealing with a specific disease, is often divided in the phases that follow:

- Primary prevention, that can be affected by AI through the use of big data, cloud systems and epidemiological patterns analysis,
- Secondary prevention, that can benefit from telemedicine, wearables, chatbots and image recognition,
- Clinical history, that, through Artificial Intelligence and Electronical Medical Records (EMRs), is way completer and more connected than it ever was,
- Physical examination, that can, again, benefit from image recognition,
- Laboratory tests, that are improved by big data and more precise values based on clinical history and patient's physical characteristics,

- Imaging, that's probably the field that's finding the most important aids through image recognition and clinical history integration.

  That is exactly what we are doing with the iDScore, the project on which I will be writing in the next chapters.

- Diagnosis, that can be helped by telemedicine and clinical decision support.

- Therapy, where drugs are being developed through AI, the treatment is way more personal with this technology, artificial intelligences can also help to find more accurate cures through gene editing and, last but not least, AIs are also helping to develop and to perform robotic surgery.

- Health care, that is being revolutionized by digital nurses, chat bots, continuative assistance and monitoring of physical and blood values, drug dosages and video record analysis in intensive care.

  Algorithms can also calculate the death risk.

Even though it's not traditionally considered to be part of medical practice, bearing in mind professor Nante's phrase of the caterpillar, which I mentioned at the beginning of this chapter, also hospital management can be heavily improved by Artificial Intelligence, and this, to the day, is AI's most important application in the medical field.

This can be done directly, by the application of the new algorithms to the management of the financial resources, or indirectly, by providing a better organization of patients, abolition of useless exams prescription, shortening of hospital stays, etc.

As a conclusion to this first section, given the fact that history tends to repeat itself, I want to focus your attention on the opposition that MYCIN, INTERNIST-1 and CASNET have faced. MYCIN's accuracy was higher than that of the specialists it was challenging; why would a patient, except for dread, not be willing to use it?

On the other hand, if a patient decides to accept, e.g., MYCIN's diagnosis, rejecting the one of the doctors; assuming it's possible, what would the **AI's legal status** become?

Returning to the present day, Industry 4.0 technologies are being increasingly adopted in healthcare, however, their main applications mostly affect healthcare management.

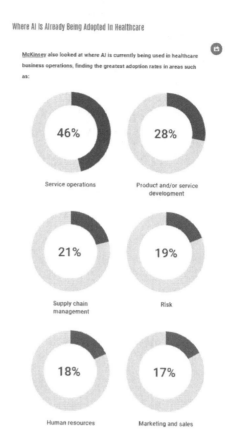

McKinsey's graph shows how the greatest AI adoption rates are found in areas such as: service operations, product and/or service development, supply chain management, risk, human resources and marketing.
This is still not enough.

The main problems that both the society and the health sector are facing, and that AIs are expected to mitigate, are the aging of the population and the consequent increase in chronic diseases and their costs.

The public health expenditure of EU members was on average 5.9% of GDP in 1990, then rising to 7.2% in 2010, and projections indicate that spending could continue to grow until 8.5% of GDP in 2060 (Eurostat).

According to what was estimated by the Digital Innovation Observatory in Healthcare of the Politecnico di Milano, the digitization of the Health System could be granting savings amounting to 6.8 billion euro per year and an overall saving for the citizens of about 7.6 billion euro (Construction of the digital public administration, 2016).

The following are considered the services with gratest saving potentials:

Healthcare Services With Greatest Cost-Saving Potential

McKinsey examined ways that AI might create more value in the business of healthcare systems and services. It estimated these potential savings at $269.4 billion annually, including:

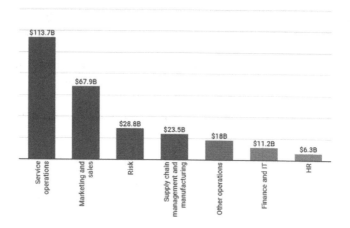

Therefore, the United Stases, among the World leaders in this field, are betting big on AIM, as shown in the following graphic:

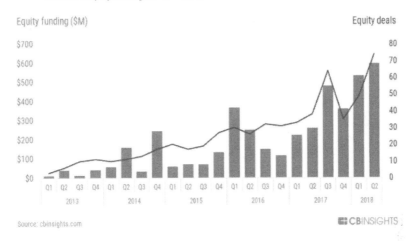

AI in healthcare funding hit a historic high in Q2'18

Disclosed equity funding, Q1'13 – Q2'18

Source: cbinsights.com

Among the many benefits that could be obtained from a conversion process towards a digital health model, the following should be considered:

- Quick and effective response to the patient's needs
- Improvement of prevention
- Enhanced management of human resources within health facilities
- Improvement of working conditions of medical personnel
- Improvement of territorial assistance
- Support for the doctor in diagnoses
- Reduced health system costs
- Democratization and decentralization of data

- Empowerment of the patient

However, for now, the only aspect of medical practice that seems to be affected by the use of these technologies is above all, if not solely, the managerial side, wasting a great part of AI's potential.

In the other fields, as we have seen in the previous chapter, "Artificial Intelligence in the World", Artificial Intelligence is much more rooted, employed, and less feared, almost replacing the working figures that it was originally supposed to assist.

The following section of this chapter will present the main examples of possible AI use in healthcare, besides managerial employement.

2.2 – Some examples of AI in Medicine

In this section of my thesis, I will write about some of the possible applications of Artificial Intelligences in the medical field.

My reflection started when I was attending the third year of Medical School, when, in Genetics class, the professor explained us the problems concerning the understanding of the human genome.

We thought they were linked to the inability to sequence the human DNA, instead, the professor told us: *"We know how to sequence the human DNA.* - The Human Genome Project (HGP) was declared complete in 2003 (genome.gov) - *We have known it for many years. What we don't know is how to read it; DNA contains an enormous quantity of data, and we don't know which ones are important and which are not."*

This posed a very significant problem for the medical field: the problem of Big Data.

Looking for a solution to this problem, I came across the American company Illumina.

Illumina, Inc. is a company incorporated in April 1998 that develops, manufactures and markets integrated systems for the analysis of genetic variation and biological function.

I bought some shares of this company too, so that I could follow more closely their management of the incredible amount of data contained in human DNA.

This is, indeed, one of the most important areas in which machines differ from human beings: the ability to manage and process a massive amount of information, finding links and correlations between extremely inhomogeneous and complex data; data that a human mind alone can't even store.

Big Data in Healthcare

"Big Data in Health refers to large routinely or automatically collected datasets, which are electronically captured and stored. It is reusable in the sense of multipurpose data and comprises the fusion and connection of existing databases for the purpose of improving health and health system performance."
European Commission, 2016

Big Data is a field that studies possible approaches to analyze and systematically extract information from data sets that are too large or complex to be processed by traditional data-processing application software.

As in the case of AI with the AI effect, presented above, also in this circumstance the definition has not an absolute value:

"For some organizations, facing hundreds of gigabytes of data for the first time may trigger a need to reconsider data management options. For others, it may take tens or hundreds of terabytes before data size becomes a significant consideration."
(Magoulas & Lorica, February 2009)

Big data, on of the founding pillars of **Industry 4.0**, is definied through the following carachteristics:

- Volume: defined as the amount of collected and stored data. The extent of the data determines the value and potential insight, and whether it can be classified as big data or not.
- Variety: the nature and the type of data collected. Big data are drawn from text, images, audios and videos, and missing information can be completed through data fusion.

- Velocity: the rate at which bid data are produced, stored and processed. Also, the speed at which they are available; big data are often collected continuously, such as through wearables, and are available in real-time.
- Veracity: the quantity of noise present in the data. The quality of data can vary greatly, affecting the accuracy of the analysis.

  As we have seen, in the medical world, the veracity can be particularly low, due to the subjectivity of both the patient and of the doctor, and the nature of their relationship.

The veracity of the medical data, in comparison to the one of data derived from other scientific fields, is considered to be lower, and this is one of the main differences between the medical word and other areas of knowledge.

Some examples of new intelligent aggregators of data collected in a dematerialized form in the health sector are the Electronic Health Record, the Assisted Notebook, the Health Dossier and the Cup 4.0 systems.

These data are different from the ones that have been collected in the past, in two ways:

- These data are **digital native**: they are not transcribed or acquired in order to make them digital (task that Amazon, trough AI is trying to do with millions of papery clinical records), but there is specific software for their acquisition and integration.

-   These data are **patient centered**: in the past, data were acquired for economic-administrative purpose, leaving the individuality of the patient in the background, big data instead are acquired in a way that the health of the single patient is put in foreground.

This second point is very important for my thesis and for AI's future perspective: as we will see in the next chapters, even in a boarder sense, client/patient profiling plays a central role in the development of new technologies and business models.

Big data, in fact, give an important contribution to one of the newest and most important frontiers of medicine: **precision medicine**, often colloquially called "tailored medicine" or "customized medicine" by our professors, in order to further emphasize how the focus of the doctor is no longer on the disease itself, but on the single patient with that disease.

In this context, the analysis of the genetic, epigenetic and transcriptional characteristics of the patient is fundamental to restructure the therapies and to change the course of pathologies which, to the day, don't have a cure.

Another important aspect regarding this issue is the fact that big data, being easily available for the patient, who, for example, can consult them directly via their smartphone or laptop, encourages an empowerment of the figure of the patient and a democratization, albeit partial, of information that was once only in the hands of the doctor (Moruzzi et al., 2018).

Technologies like this, if used in all the hospitals, thing that unfortunately does not happen, could make us forget the question that all patients are asked as soon as they enter the clinic: *"Did you bring the sheets of the last visits with you?"*.

This data, in fact, would not need to be transported manually, nor to be saved in a digital oblivion that nobody consults, nor to be read in full: the results, in fact, would be presented in real time by the analysis made by the AI which is at the base of these systems.

In fact, no one cares about knowing whether a given value is 10, 20 or 100, what matters is whether the value is considered high, low, or normal, and whether it is increased or decreased, for that specific patient, of that specific family, of that specific community.

This can be done in a rudimentary and gross way by a doctor who, manually, frenetically consults anachronistic written deeds, or infallibly and instantaneously from a machine that knows the same data of all the patients of a city, of a Region, or of the whole World.

Who would do it better?

Above all, who is doing it right now in our hospitals?

Wearables

Remaining in the vast field of big data, this section will briefly present the hardware devices that favor their collection and that, through cloud platforms and artificial intelligence, provide an almost immediate analysis.

Wearables are smart electronic devices that can be incorporated into clothing or worn on the body as implants or accessories. They are an example of **Internet of Things**: object that exchange information through the internet without the direct interaction or input of humans.

Wearables popularity grew enormously with the introduction of the smartwatch (above all: Samsung Galaxy Gear, September 2013, and Apple Watch, April 2015) and, after that, the one of the fitness trackers.

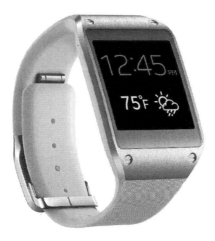

Samsung Galaxy Gear

According to CCS Insight, healthcare wearables market is going to be worth $34.2 billion by 2020 (as shown in the picture below) and, according to Juniper Research, it will reach $60 billion by 2023.

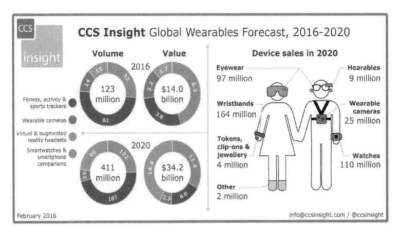

(Forbes, 2016)

Wearable technology is classically divided into the following categories:

- Sport and fitness, referring to wearables mainly used for secondary prevention.
- Treatment monitoring, such as in the case of patients suffering from chronical diseases, e.g.: diabetes, that need continuous cures and one-to-one care

Wearables can be used to collect information on a user's healthiness, including:

- Time spent exercising
- Calories consumed

- Steps walked
- Heart rate
- Blood pressure
- Sleeping habits
- Release of biochemicals

Currently other applications within healthcare are being studied, such as:

- Measuring blood alcohol content (Greathouse, 2017)
- Measuring athletic performance (Bell, 2017)
- Long-term monitoring of patients with heart and circulatory problems that records an electrocardiogram and is self-moistening,
- Health Risk Assessment applications, including measures of frailty and risks of age-dependent diseases (Tim Pyrkov, 2018)
- Detecting breast cancer (Cyrcadia Health's iTBra),
- Temperature tracking (TempTraq)

However, the great advantages brought by this technology, that will be illustrated in the next sections of this script (e.g.: personalization, early diagnosis, remote patient monitoring, adherence to medication, information registry, optimum decision by the doctor, healthcare cost savings) are accompanied by many controversies.

Above all, a patient who is using a Samsung wearable in order to monitor, for example, his sleep, can ask himself: "What will Samsung do with my data?".

This question introduces two of the biggest problems concerning big data and wearables: **privacy** and **processing of sensitive data**.

Imaging

The specialist that will face the biggest threat posed by artificial intelligence algorithms is, without any doubt, the one that is more related to image recognition: Radiology.

"AI's impact will be monumental—will radiologists go along for the ride or be left in the dust?"
Dave Pearson, October 2017, Radiology Business

Its main applications include:

- Computer-aided diagnosis,
- Clinical decision support
- Quantitative analysis tools
- Computer-aided detection

A recent example of AI's capabilities could be the one of the commercial artificial intelligence system that matched the accuracy of over 28,000 interpretations of breast cancer screening mammograms by 101 radiologists (Rodriguez- Ruiz et al., March 2019).

Another example is the one of a study at Stanford that created an algorithm that could spot pneumonia at the exact site, in those patients involved, with a better average F1 metric (a statistical metric based on accuracy and recall), than the radiologists included in that trial.

Artificial Intelligence also outperforms human specialists in a lot of other fields, such as: echocardiography (Strickland, 2018), thyroid nodules mangement (Mateusz Buda, July 9, 2019), prostate cancer (Cao, Bajgiran, Mirak, & al., 2019) and brain aneurysms detection (Stanford University, June 2019), just to cite a few.

In terms of revenue, global Artificial Intelligence radiology market was valued at US$ 187.61 million in 2018 and is anticipated to reach US$ 3506.55 million by 2027, growing at a CAGR of 16.5% over the forecast period (Market Insights, July 2019).

Even in this field, specialists fear AI and are skeptical about its absolute dominance in comparison to trained radiologist.

Their position is synthesized into 6 points by PhD Maciej A.Mazurowski, author of "Artificial Intelligence may cause a significant disruption to the radiology workforce":

- AI will never be able to match radiologists' performance;
- radiologists do more than interpret images;
- even if AI takes over a large portion of the reading tasks, the radiologists' effort will be shifted toward interactions with patients and other physicians;
- the FDA would never agree to let machines do the work of radiologist;
- the issues of legal liability would be insurmountable; and
- patients would never put complete trust in computer algorithms.

The author concludes that the readiologists' believes are true – for now.

The near future, however, is ready to crush their certainties and in the radiology community, as well as in the medical one, "an honest, in-depth discussion is needed to guide development of the field."

Drugs and vaccines

The feedback-driven drug development process starts from existing results obtained from numerous sources such as high-throughput compound and fragment screening, computational modelling and data available in literature. The procedure alternates induction and deduction fases and this cycle eventually leads to optimised hit and lead compounds. Automation of specific parts of the cycle reduces randomness and errors and improves the efficiency of drug development.

De novo design approaches require knowledge of organic chemistry for in silico compound synthesis and virtual screening models that function as surrogates for biochemical and biological tests of efficacy.

Eventually, active learning algorithms allow the identification of new compounds with promising activities against a given target.

The technologies that incorporate AI can be applied in various stages of drug development, such as: target identification, drug design and repurposing, R&D improving, refinition of the decision-making process to recruit patients for clinical trials, pharmacological properties studies, protein characteristics, drug combination and drug–target association, identification of new pathways and targets using omics analysis, etc.

According to some estimations, main drugmakers spend more than $2.5 billion to get a new medicine to patients. In fact, just 1 out of 10 therapies that enters human trials makes it to the market. And **science moves slowly**: In the nearly 20 years since the human genome was sequenced, researchers have discovered treatments for a tiny fraction of the approximately 7000 known rare diseases.

Furthermore, there are roughly 20000 genes that can malfunction in at least 100000 ways, and millions of possible interactions between the resulting proteins. It's unbearable for drugmakers to examinate all of those combinations by hand (Langreth, July 2019).

"If we want to understand the other 97 percent of human biology, we will have to acknowledge it is too complex for humans."

Chris Gibson, Recursion Pharmaceuticals co-founder and CEO

An important part of drug development consist in predicting the shapes that proteins will acquire when synthesized, since they are the building blocks of both cells and drugs and there are more possible protein shapes than there are atoms in the universe.

And this is where **DeepMind** enters the scene.

DeepMind Technologies is a British artificial intelligence company founded in September 2010, acquired by Google in 2014, and currently owned by Alphabet Inc.

Having laid waist to Atari classics and reached superhuman performances both in chess and in Chinese board game Go, Google's DeepMind, that has also been mentioned in the first chapter of this script, turned his renowned artificial intelligence on protein shapes.

As a result, in December 2018, at the CASP13 meeting in Riviera Maya, Mexico, DeepMind beat experienced biologists at predicting the shapes of proteins, in a result that was described as "absolutely stunning" and "a total surprise" by scientists that partook to the event.

An important disclaimer made by DeepMind's researches was that their technology's aim was *not* to replace scientists of pharmacists, but to help them in the medicine-discovery process.

Why did they specify it?

Also social-media giant **Facebook Inc.**, which silently released a paper using AI (Alexander Rives, 2019) to analyze 250 million protein sequences in April, is taking part in this race, giving Big Pharma a run for its money (Langreth, July 2019).

Given the potential of this new disruptive application of Artificial Intelligence, Big Pharma is closing new deals with companies that are specialized in its development, as shown in the following graph.

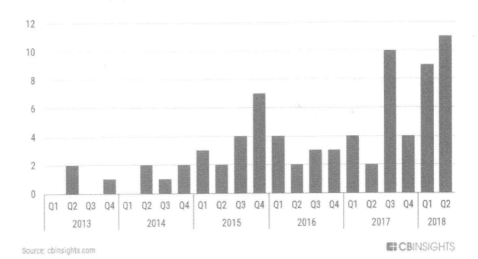

The images shows the growing interest of pharmaceutical companies through the years.

Regarding **vaccines**, however, it is news of a few days ago that Australian researchers have just released the World's first AI-developed vaccine.

An AI called SAM (Search Algorithm for Ligands), developed by Flinders University Professor Nikolai Petrovsky was able, for the first time in history, to independently create an influenza vaccine.

Petrovsky said that the use of AIs such as SAM potentially shortens the normal drug discovery and development process by decades and saves hundreds of millions of dollars (Masige, July 2019).

Resuming DeepMind's researchers words about the role of artificial intelligence in helping scientists to discover new drugs, and not in replacing them to accomplish that task, are we still sure that this isn't going to happen?

If it were possible that this would happen, would it be more important to give scientists a job or to discover new drugs?

Another concern regards the role of tech companies if they were to gain the market share that now belongs to Big Pharma: what kind of corporation would they become?

Robotics in Healthcare

Also in the form of robots, AI is shaping up Medicine, and these are some of its main applications:

- Robot Assisted Surgery: it's not a new technology, what's new is the fact that, trough always more complex AI based alorithms, surgery is becoming more and more precise, reducing sequelae, complications and duration of hospital stays. Slowly, robots are also acquiring a crescent degree of freedom from human supervision.
- Clinical Training Bots: important for surgical practice and able to respond in real time to the specialists' actions.
- Companion and psychological support bots: in form of physical robots, voice assistants and chatbots, are able to assist the patient and to detect suicidal risk
- Robotic nurses: robotic assistants that can handle digital paperwork, take measurements of vital signs, monitor patient's conditions, moving carts and gurneys from a room to another or even drawing blood

(Tomlinson, 2018)

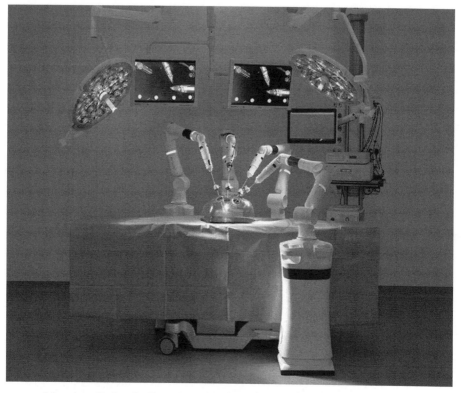

Versius Robotic Surgical System (MedGadget,2018)

It goes without saying that even the robotic surgeons have been greeted by **strong criticisms**, and, to the day, are still considered shiny machines that are not often used (Datteri, 2009).

At this point of my script, what I hope that readers are wondering is: why are these technologies, if they are so effective, not adopted in clinical practice? Why are them always greeted by all these criticisms? Why is it so only in the medical world?

The next chapter will give answers to these questions.

*"The greatest enemy of knowledge is not ignorance; it is the
illusion of knowledge."*
Attributed to Stephen W. Hawking

Chapter 3.

Clash or convergence?

Taking up the questions and considerations with which the
previous chapter ended, it is important to note that artificial
intelligences, although often considered in the collective
imagination as such futuristic technologies as to find no practical
application, are actually currently widely used in many industries
and in many sectors.

We have also to keep in mind Raymond Kurzweil's theories,
presented in the first chapter, that are a key point in
understanding the urgency and the importance of discussing
these topics.

In the medical field, however, as we have seen, the situation is very different. This is due to several reasons, which will be discussed in the next sections.

The first concerns the **technologies themselves**: it is true that they have thousands of merits and that they bring many advantages, but, like every invention, they also bring risks and negative repercussions. However, even the invention of fire has brought with it the risk of arsons.

The second concerns the **medical class**, which, especially in Italy, is elderly and is therefore devoid of a digital culture that allows it to know and to understand these technologies, and therefore make use of them.
In this regard, I will also talk about my experience in the dermatology department during this academic year.
Just to give an example, a doctor refused to acquire the dermoscopic images of some patients simply because she was not able to use the software depleted.

The third concerns the **relationship** between the two figures of this clash: technologies still have great limitations, and the medical class is not prepared to face nor to overcome them, but it is also true that the medical field, unlike many others, is much more particular.
This point, of particular importance, will be further deepened in the next chapter.

The doctors in fact do not have to deal only with numbers or needs that are easy to manage, but with people, wounded, sick and scared, to whom doctors must understand the illness, the physical aspect and the psychological aspect, without neglecting the "human side" of the problem.

However, the rhetoric of the "human side" is often used by the medical class to hide its limitations and its inability or unwillingness to learn new and different concepts, which are often far beyond their preparation.

In Italy, as we will see, these problems are even aggravated by the social, demographic and cultural situation in which the Country finds itself.

The next chapters, instead, include a possible solution to some of the problems presented in the following sections and is about my personal experience in the application of the iDScore platform, developed by Professor Cevenini et al., in the Dermatology Department of Siena, led by Professor Rubegni.

3.1 – Problems concerning artificial intelligence in healthcare

In addition to countless and enormous advantages, artificial intelligence also presents some limitations, which means that there are doubts about its use, especially in the medical field.

One of the first mentioned limits concerns the functioning of this technology, in fact, **artificial intelligences are black boxes**.

As in a black box of a plane, we know that artificial intelligences have an input, the data that are given to them, and an output, the results and the solutions that the algorithms are asked to find.

It's known that a program written by a human is run, but we don't know how it works and, mostly, the algorithm isn't able to explain, or even show, the process that led it to the problem's solution (Bathaee, Spring 2018).

Thus presented, the black box problem may seem insurmountable, and can lead doctors and patients to fear artificial intelligences and their functioning, and that's what's happening.

The question, however, can be differently approached. For instance, every day, doctors prescribe hundreds of drugs, but many of them do not know how they work. Not because of their negligence, but, simply, as in the case of acetylsalicylic acid, because nobody knows its exact operating mechanism (London, February 2019).

The same discourse can also be applied to the "clinical sense" or to the intuition of a doctor who, at first sight, recognizes the pathology of a patient, without being able to explain precisely the reasons that led him to its conclusion.

It is true that, on a philosophical level, the problem of black boxes is a very multifaceted and elaborate one, but, more generally, if a person were to use only tools whose functioning is perfectly well known, he would probably not use either the car, nor the telephone, nor the computer.

In conclusion, as **Aristotle** noted over two millennia ago, when our knowledge of causal systems is incomplete and precarious, the ability to explain how results are produced can be less important than the ability to produce such results and empirically verify their accuracy (London, February 2019).

Another important issue is the one regarding **privacy and personal data treatment**.

Data security is the priority for healthcare organizations, especially in the wake of a rapid-fire series of high-profile breaches, hackings, and ransomware episodes, that also affected many tech firms, with special reference to Zuckerberg-owned social media companies (Facebook, Instagram and WhatsApp).

Recently, the problem of the data supplied to the FaceApp aging application has been widely discussed, as well as, months before, Facebook's 10 years challenge: in both cases, users have voluntarily provided the social media giants with pictures of their faces, described by hashtags, that can be easily analyzed, and related to the login data that need to be submitted in order to sign in.

Back to medical practice, from phishing attacks to malware to laptops accidentally left in a cab, healthcare data is subject to a nearly infinite array of vulnerabilities.

The HIPAA Security Rule comprises a long list of technical safeguards for administrations storing protected health information (PHI), including transmission security, authentication protocols, and controls over access, integrity, and auditing.

In practice, these precautions translate into common-sense security actions such as using up-to-date anti-virus software, setting up firewalls, encrypting sensitive data, and using multi-factor authentication.

But even the most firmly secured data center can be taken down by the fallibility of human staff members, who tend to prioritize convenience over lengthy software updates and complicated constraints on their access to data or software.

Healthcare organizations must regularly remind their staff members of the critical nature of data security protocols and consistently review who has access to high-value data assets to avoid malicious parties from causing harm (Bresnick, 2017).

Another issue is the one affecting **anonymization**: with so much data, it could become impossible to completely remove the ability to identify an individual; the problem is known as *"The Mosaic Effect"* (Mazmanian, 2014).
This also relates to the fact that **big data will probably exist forever**: in the past, papery clinical data were lost to arhieves renoval and digital ones were a lot fewer and more frammentary, and softwares weren't able to analyze them entirely in order to relate them to their owner.

One more important knot is the one concerning **bias**.
In addition to programming-related problems, there is the fact that Artificial Intelligence, to this day, is still often limited by the natural intelligence that created it and by the data fed to the algorithms.

For instance, vision algorithms trained on unbalanced data sets failed to recognize women or people of color; hiring programs fed historic data were proven to perpetuate discrimination that already exists (Hao, 2019).

Tied to the issue of bias – and harder to fix – is the **lack of diversity across the AI field** itself. Women occupy, at most, 30% of industry jobs and fewer than 25% of teaching roles at top universities. There are comparatively few black and Latin researchers as well (Hao, 2019).

This shows that, provided that artificial intelligence will depend on natural intelligence, it will present most of the limits that characterize the human mind and behaviors.
Other problems will rise when Artificial Intelligence, overcome the human one, will be completely independent from it.

The last of the *tangible* problems, but probably the first in importance, is that concerning **unemployment** and its management.

Although Robert Gordon, like most economists, sees it as a positive fact, it is undeniable that many jobs will be lost due to automation.
As soon as in 2017, McKinsey Research reported that up to one-third of U.S. workers — and 800 million globally — could be

displaced by 2030 and that "60 percent of occupations have at least 30 percent of constituent work activities that could be automated" (Franck, 2017).

Also, according to analysis firm Oxford Economics 2019 report, up to 20 million manufacturing jobs around the world could be replaced by robots by 2030 (Cellan-Jones, June 2019).

The source also described the change in the use of robots between 2011 and 2016.

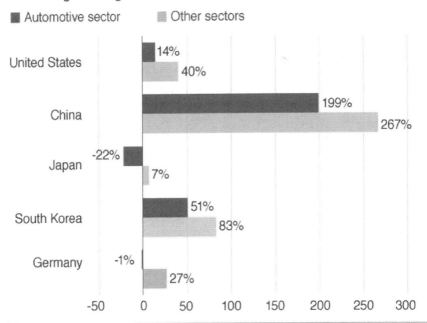

The rise of the robots

Percentage change in the use of robots between 2011 and 2016

■ Automotive sector   ▨ Other sectors

United States
14%
40%

China
199%
267%

Japan
-22%
7%

South Korea
51%
83%

Germany
-1%
27%

-50   0   50   100   150   200   250   300

Source: Oxford Economics   BBC

The graph underlines how China, as seen in the healthcare section, is the World leader in the Artificial Intelligence technological revolution.

In addition to it, Oxford Economics lists the countries that experienced more job losses since 2000. It will not be a surprise to find out who is in first place in this ranking.

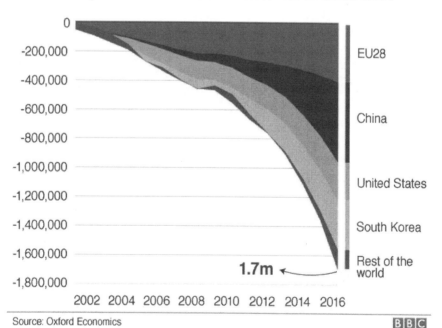

Where most jobs have been lost
Cumulative job losses attributed to automation since 2000

Source: Oxford Economics

China, in fact, lost more than half a billion jobs, compared to 400000 in Europe and 260000 in the United States (Cellan-Jones, June 2019).

The firm concludes its research by saying that, at a global level, jobs will be created at the rate they are destroyed, so, in their view, the only problem will be to train and relocate the workers left unemployed.
Will doctors also face this issue?

The last fear concerns the **existential risk** posed by Artificial General Intelligence, AGI.
Artificial General Intelligence (AGI) is the intelligence of a machine that can do any task a human can do, while Super Intelligence (SI) is an agent whose abilities far surpass the brightest and most gifted human minds.

"Hope we're not just the biological boot loader for digital superintelligence. Unfortunately, that is increasingly probable"
Elon Musk

Even if the topic is still widely debated, many of the AI experts, such as Raymond Kurzweil, Bill Gates, Stephen Hawking and Elon Musk fear that, once a machine gained an intelligence similar to the human one, in few months it can reach Super Intelligence, posing a threat to mankind (Parkin, 2018).

Let's say that an AI researcher creates a program able to reach his intelligence and programming capability: once the Artificial Intelligence reached his level, it could rewrite itself in order to surpass it.

The second-generation AI could do the same thing, but in about half of the time, and so on. From generation to generation, this AIs can become always more intelligent and this can be done every time a lot faster (Parkin, 2018).

It's the same approach that AlphaGo Zero used in order to become the greatest Go player of the World in 2017.

The World, however, seems not to be worried about this scenario, as stated by Stephen Hawking in 2014.

"So, facing possible futures of incalculable benefits and risks, the experts are surely doing everything possible to ensure the best outcome, right? Wrong. If a superior alien civilization sent us a message saying, 'We'll arrive in a few decades,' would we just reply, 'OK, call us when you get here—we'll leave the lights

on?' Probably not–but this is more or less what is happening
with AI."

Stephen Hawking, 2014.

And there are also many experts, such as Mark Zuckerberg and Facebook Chief AI Scientist and 2018 Turing Award winner **Yann LeCun**, who argue that super intelligent machines will have no desire for self-preservation (Dowd, 2017).

This topic, of particular importance, will be taken up again and deepened in the last chapter of the paper.

For now, what is central is to emphasize that, although artificial intelligences have an almost unlimited potential, the risks that they pose are also considerable, and must be kept in mind.

At this point, one might ask why no one in the medical field discusses the aforementioned problems.
The answer to the question is found in the next section: Medical Class limits.

3.2 – Medical Class limits

"When Henry Ford made cheap, reliable cars, people said: 'Nah, what's wrong with a horse?'"
Elon Musk

As defined, couples are made by two figures and, if it is true that artificial intelligences have their limits, it is also true that even the medical profession has given good reasons for not making the relationship with the new technologies work.

One of the characteristics of the medical class, in Italy, is **oldness**.

The average age of hospital and ASL health personnel is now 51 years old.

The medical and technical-professional staff is close to the average of 53 years, surpassed by the management staff that with 53.4 years is the oldest and aged group since 2010, when the average age was 49.7 years (Centro Studi Nebo, May 2019).

As a consequence of this condition, doctors not only did not receive an adequate computer training (for example, almost all doctors do not know how to code), but also they no longer have either the mental elasticity, nor, even less, the will to learn how to use the new technologies.

In addition to this, a 2016 study found that physicians spent about two hours doing computer work for every hour spent face to face with a patient; this means that two thirds of the work that a doctor does is devoted to activities that require the use of the computer, and this condition has, as we will see, serious implications (Gawande, November 2018).

In my personal experience in Dermatology Department, I also noticed the fact that few minutes were, de facto, spent for the visit of the patient itself, while many more for the check in, for the writing of the clinical data on the paper that also contains the diagnosis and that is given to the patient at the end of the visit, and for the procedures relating to the payment of the ticket.

In fact, in the clinic that I used to attend to, a doctor visited the patient, while another, sitting for the whole time in front of the computer, continuously filled in all the necessary forms necessary for the visit, and, while the visit itself could be a pleasant activity, filling out all the forms was stressful and **frustrating**, since the doctors didn't always know how to use the platform properly, and the platform was not designed to meet their needs.

Also, going back to the aforementioned study, it pointed that, in the examination room, physicians devoted half of their patient time facing the screen to do electronic tasks. And these tasks were spilling over after hours. The University of Wisconsin found that the average workday for its family physicians had grown to eleven and a half hours (Gawande, November 2018).
The result has been epidemic levels of **burnout** among clinicians. Forty per cent screen positive for **depression**, and seven per cent report **suicidal thinking**—almost double the rate of the general working population. The number of doctor suicides – 28 to 40 per 100000 – is also more than twice that of the other professions (Gawande, November 2018).

Medscape, in January 2019, also pointed out the main reasons that concurred in doctor's burnout, finding out that bureaucratic tasks, that often involve the use of PCs, and the computerization itself of clinical practice are two of the main reasons for this pathology to occur (Kane, Jan 2019).

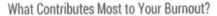

What Contributes Most to Your Burnout?

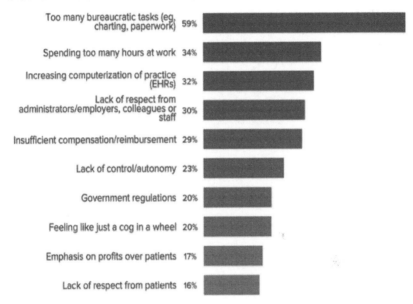

Too many bureaucratic tasks (eg, charting, paperwork)	59%
Spending too many hours at work	34%
Increasing computerization of practice (EHRs)	32%
Lack of respect from administrators/employers, colleagues or staff	30%
Insufficient compensation/reimbursement	29%
Lack of control/autonomy	23%
Government regulations	20%
Feeling like just a cog in a wheel	20%
Emphasis on profits over patients	17%
Lack of respect from patients	16%

Since the relationship that the medical world has with computers is so troubled and conflicting, we cannot expect the one with artificial intelligences to be different, even simply because doctors don't know what these new technologies are and what they are capable of.

Doctors think that artificial intelligences are just more powerful software than they already have, instead, AIs can be a more powerful *mind* than they already have.

However, as said, age, lack of training, inertia, and the troubled relationship they have with technology leads them to greatly **underestimate the benefit** they could derive from these inventions.

The opinions of two doctors about the use of artificial intelligences will be brought as an example.

The first is doctor Lallas, Department of Dermatology and Venereology, Aristotle University, Thessaloniki, Greece, that in a 2018 study titled "Artificial intelligence and melanoma diagnosis: ignoring human nature may lead to false predictions" concluded that:

"Humans like to interact with humans, in general, and even more in medicine. The moment that a physician examines a patient is a unique interaction during which a human being uses all available knowledge and mental effort to help another human being. There is a lot of interchange of energy in this procedure. This is very much superior to a simple judgment on the benign or malignant nature of a lesion. The result of a medical consultation is not measured only by the absolute improvement of the patient's physical health. Think for a moment about

patients with end-stage metastatic cancer, those not responsive to treatment, or patients with diseases with no available treatments. They build a strong relationship with their doctor, which is not measurable or explainable by the absolute improvement of their physical health. To think that medical care can be simply conducted by mathematical models is tantamount to ignoring human nature."

This is *exactly* why I am writing this thesis. This is *precisely* what I want to fight against.

Doctors Lallas and Argenziano, in these few lines, have brought the experience of millions of doctors around the world.

They have shown, in fact, that they have no idea of what an Artificial Intelligence is and of how it can be applied to clinical practice.

If they think that a *faster* diagnosis or that an instrument that can help them make that diagnosis will take away from them the "interchange of energy" with their patients, they also show that they do not have a single clue of what these new technologies are for.

If, on the other hand, we think that, little by little, these technologies can replace doctors, wouldn't that also mean that clinicians will have an increasing amount of time to spend with their patients?

Before that, how could a faster and more accurate diagnosis make a doctor waste his time?

In my humble opinion, anachronistic, alchemical and witchcraft conceptions like those of the *"interchange of energy"* are nothing more than brisk rhetoric aimed at concealing one's own ignorance.

Moreover, if a doctor wants to spend quality time with a patient in order to create a strong and significative bond, it will certainly not be a computer, nor a robot, to stop him.

Historically, new technologies and changes in society have always been blamed for the loss of values, of **"mos maiorum"**, but I am deeply convinced that values are lost only by people who never really had them.

The second example is the one involving Dr. Eric Topol, author of "Deep Medicine: How Artificial Intelligence Can Make Healthcare Human Again" (2019).

In his book, he claims the opposite of what Doctor Lallas and Doctor Argenziano are convinced of.

Dr. Topol, in fact, is persuaded that by automating clinical practices using Artificial Intelligence, the doctors can again have time to devote to their patients.

In an interview to The New York Times he stated:

"What I'm most excited about is using the future to bring back the past: to restore the care in health care. By giving both the gift of time to clinicians, who are at peak levels ever recorded for burnout and depression, and empowerment to patients, for those who want it, this will ultimately be possible. But it will require substantial activism of the medical community to stand up for patients and not allow the jump in productivity to further squeeze clinicians, upending the erosion of the doctor-patient relationship."

(O'Connor, March 2019)

He also added that, in his view, clinicians and surgeons can't and won't ever be matched or overtaken by artificial intelligences (O'Connor, March 2019).

What would these technologies be then, in his view? Mechanical secretaries? Automated stenographers? Is that it?
What's the point, then, in writing a book about them?

In this section, therefore, the limits of the medical class have been presented, which, together with the problems concerning artificial intelligences, bring the relationship between doctors and technologies to be conflicting and troublesome.

Moreover, there is a third issue, that occurs only in Medicine, which is that of the very nature of this subject: the fact that, between doctors and computers, there are people who suffer, who die, who are afraid, and this often creates further problems in the application of these new technologies.

This topic, however, will be resumed and deepened also in the next chapter.

3.3 – Current conception of Medicine

"Once we understand something, it's just maths"
Mark Zuckerberg

The peculiarity of medicine is that, as they say, *"it is not an exact science"*.

This means that, although scientific studies lead to the continuous expansion of knowledge of the doctors, there are still many dark aspects that escape the understanding of the human mind.

Moreover, one aspect is undoubtedly the fact that, when a person is sick or in danger of life, he experiences a series of feelings and emotions that distort his perception and his way of representing and describing reality.

Therefore, the doctor must understand both the disease and the patient, and *that* specific disease in *that* specific patient, and must treat them all.

In the medical world, hence, clinicians ended up wondering if Medicine has to be considered Science or Art (Panda, 2006).
In Cecil's Textbook of Medicine (Goldman and Dennis, 2004), for instance, Medicine is:

"...a profession that incorporates science and scientific methods with the art of being a physician. The art of tending to the sick is as old as humanity itself. Compared with its long and generally distinguished history of caring and comforting, the scientific basis of medicine is remarkably recent. Further the physician is advised to understand the patient as a person. Three fundamental principles are important to practitioners. They are primacy of patient welfare, patient autonomy and social justice.

The first principle lays emphasis on the patient. Patient's interest, concern or welfare comes first. The plethora of diagnoses and treatment options are secondary and subsidiary to patient welfare. The second principle speaks of the final decision about his or her treatment option, which lies with the patient. A doctor only recommends. In the process of dealing with patients, social justice again is of utmost priority. It is important because the doctor is responsible for the individual patient and to the society at large. He should ensure that health care and health services are equally accessible and available to people of all strata of society."

(Panda, 2006).

Without entering into the merits of the issue, which remains questionable, what is undoubted is that even the doctors do not know in depth the most intimate mechanisms of the human mind, nor the physiopathology of many diseases, therefore it becomes difficult for them to explain or even understand many aspects of clinical practice, from the issues regarding patients to the ones regarding illnesses.

Medicine is therefore described by many authors as an Art, and the doctor's clinical sense can be considered its brush.

A similar example, though, may be that of the thunders, which millennia ago were believed to be generated by the gods. Now that scientists have described the mechanisms of their formation, they have gone from being magic to being science.

However, as far as the brain is concerned, this process is much more complicated; as stated by Pugh's Law: *"If the human brain were simple enough to be understood by us, we would be too stupid to understand it."*

Therefore, this paradox makes us slaves of our human nature and places our own brain beyond our comprehension.

The clinical sense, thus, as well as the fact of understanding the patient and its condition, is nothing but intuition, genius, and can only be considered as Art – and not Science.

However, other aspects of this important topic will be further exposed and explained in the following chapter.

In conclusion, if understanding Medicine is tough – if not impossible – even for Human Beings, until Artificial Intelligence surpasses natural one, it will be even more difficult for it to have a chance in taking on this challenge.

It is also clear that, if AI could even just equal the human mind, it would then be able to overcome it and eventually describe it to Mankind, thus solving humanity's paradox defined by Pugh's Law.

The point of this chapter, therefore, is to describe the conflict between the medical world, partly or above all qualitative, and the technological one, purely quantitative.

To date, technologies are still limited, and even the medical world is much more complex and misunderstood than many other areas of knowledge in which the application of AI is a lot easier, however, the figure with the biggest glitches is the one of the doctor, that, not knowing and not understanding the new technologies, it fears them, and therefore it violently opposes them – or, at best, it does not make use of them, wasting a lot of money and potentially endless benefits.

As if, by sticking the eyes at this revolution and its future repercussions – of which the whole world is talking – they ceased to exist.

The next chapter, **"Industry 4.0"**, will be an introduction to the world that is approaching Medicine and its paradigms, and how healthcare is adapting and should adapt to it.

Being two worlds still very distant from each other, as shown, both must take a step in the direction of the other.

"Just as electricity transformed almost everything 100 years ago, today I actually have a hard time thinking of an industry that I don't think AI will transform in the next several years."

(Ng, 2017).

Chapter 4.

Healthcare 4.0

The fourth chapter of my paper will be focused on Industry 4.0.

Industry 4.0, as explained in the next section, is given by the set of technologies that fall into, but are not limited only to, the incredibly vast field of Artificial Intelligence.

Industry 4.0 Revolution will be different from all the other industrial revolutions that humanity has faced, as well as the technologies that underlie it are different from every other technology ever created by Humanity, both in form and in substance.

Specifically, however, and in the merits of this thesis, we must also underline the fact that clinical practice, due to its peculiarities, is completely different from all the other areas to which the paradigms of the next industrial revolution can be applied, as we have begun to see in the previous section of this paper.

If it is true that both the technologies and, above all, the medical class have their faults, as we have seen in the previous chapter, it is also true that the playing field on which they collide (or meet) has particularities that make it unique, and that must be evaluated carefully to ensure that AI can be a benefit, and not a damage, to clinical practice.

The peculiar characteristics of the health sector will be exposed below, following the definition and the presentation of Industry 4.0.
The last part of this chapter, merging its first two sections, will be focused on Healthcare 4.0: the application of the fourth industrial revolution paradigm to clinical practice.

4.1 – The fourth industrial revolution – Industry 4.0

The term Industry 4.0 is used to define what today is identified as the "Fourth Industrial Revolution" that – unlike the previous ones – does not arise as a result of radical changes in the productive fabric linked to the introduction of a single technology, but rather comes from integration of different new technologies that do not individually represent breaking elements, but that collectively and through their interactions manage to trigger a revolutionary change.

In particular, there are three aspects that make this revolution different from those that have occurred so far: speed, scope and intensity, and impact on systems (Schwab 2016):

1. **Speed**: previous industrial revolutions occurred at a linear speed, while the current one presents an **exponential** speed of growth and this finds its foundation in the heterogeneous nature of the world in which we live which is constantly interconnected, and in the fact that existing technologies create new and ever better ones;

2. **Scope and intensity**: the transformation is based on the digital revolution and combines different technologies, giving rise to unprecedented paradigm shifts at individual, economic, corporate and social level.

3. **The impact on systems**: this revolution involves and transforms entire systems, countries, companies, sectors and societies in general.

This revolution relies on four fundamental pillars such as Internet of Things, Cloud Computing, Big Data Analytics and advanced technologies such as artificial intelligence, sensors, robots and 3D printing that impact on companies at the level of:

- Product: changing the way of design and develop the products/services offered;
- Process: modifying the management of the distribution chain;
- Customer: allowing the customer's needs to be analyzed in greater depth for better customer satisfaction.

A definition of Industry 4.0 is provided by M. Hermann (et al., 2015) in "Design principles for Industrie 4.0 scenarios":

"Industry 4.0 is a collective term for technologies and concepts of value chain organization. Within the modular Smart Factories of Industry 4.0, Cyber Physical System monitor physical

processes, create virtual physical and make decentralized decisions. Over the Internet of Things, Cyber Physical System communicate and cooperate with each other and humans in real time. Via the Internet of Service, both internal and cross-organizational services are offered and utilized by participants of the value chain."

These technologies, if taken individually, cannot overturn industrial processes, but, if integrated together, they are able to make three fundamental activities possible with revolutionary effects on production and consumption (Giacomo Assenza et al., 2018):

1. The ability to measure, therefore, to collect and store large amounts of **data**. Nowadays devices such as chips, sensors and transmitters are incorporated into industrial components and allow data to be constantly detected.

2. The ability to communicate and share this data in **real time**. In industry 4.0, devices are not only able to detect large amounts of data, but with the use of standardized protocols they can also transmit and integrate them with other systems and assets, creating an intense and continuous flow of communication.

3. The ability to **infer**, therefore, to analyze complex data quickly, drawing useful information to support the decision-making process.

In recent Deloitte "Forces of change" report it is emphasized that the concept of Industry 4.0 is mainly based on a cyclical process whose motor is the continuous flow of information and data processed through actions resulting from the interaction between physical reality and the world digital.

To obtain this process, the different technologies must be integrated together in order to be able to increase a cycle of three phases:

1. **Physical to digital**: represents the first phase, in which it is necessary to collect data from the physical world and digitize them so as to make them usable by the various electronic devices.

2. **Digital to digital**: represents the second phase, and consists in the communication and processing of data in real time by the set of advanced technologies that are connected to each other.

3. **Digital to physical**: this last step represents the moment of closure of the cycle in which, through appropriate algorithms and automation processes, the decisions elaborated by the digital world can

materialize into actions and changes within the physical world.

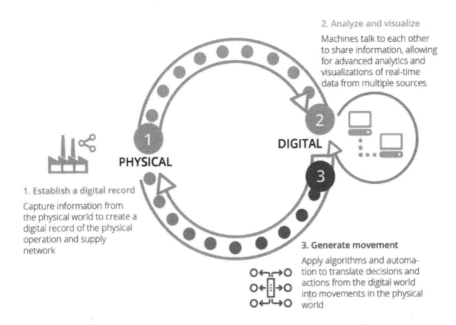

2. Analyze and visualize

Machines talk to each other to share information, allowing for advanced analytics and visualizations of real-time data from multiple sources

DIGITAL

PHYSICAL

1. Establish a digital record

Capture information from the physical world to create a digital record of the physical operation and supply network

3. Generate movement

Apply algorithms and automa-tion to translate decisions and actions from the digital world into movements in the physical world

This paradigm is being exported also to the medical world, creating what it's known as "**Healthcare 4.0**"; the iDScore is a practical example of the application of this model and, as such, represents one of the first conscious steps towards the healthcare revolution.

However, before presenting Healthcare 4.0 and the iDScore, the next section of this chapter will focus on the specific features that make the health sector unique and that must be kept in mind in order to develop a technology suited to its peculiarity.

4.2 – The specific features of the health sector

"Digital technology is an intrinsic part of almost every area of life. How can we ensure that developments in this field, especially those that rely on artificial intelligence (AI), meet all our ethical, legal and technological concerns?"
(Medica, July 2019)

In the previous chapter we have highlighted how the medical class, nowadays, especially in Italy, presents great intrinsic limits that restrict their understanding, first, and then their adoption of the new technologies.

The doctors, as demonstrated, are elderly, and therefore have not had adequate training for the adoption of artificial intelligences.

This means that, often, by demonizing them, they cause depressive or burn-out phenomena in them and this, in turn, creates a vicious circle that does nothing more than increase doctors' fear of new technologies and therefore reduce their study and use.

It has also been shown that, due to their training, doctors tend to have an anachronistic conception of medicine, which leads them to demonize and fear new discoveries, taking refuge in the obsolete practice that they learned decades earlier.

In my opinion, this aspect is the main fault of the late adoption of artificial intelligences in clinical practice, and, even if it were not, it would still be a mortal sin for a man of science to fear formation and knowledge.

This being said, it is necessary to give the medical class credit for having at least two justifications: the first, as we have seen at the end of the previous chapter, is that clinical practice is a **particular** branch of the sciences, and, as such, it is difficult to define and therefore to change or improve it, also through AI.

The second is that, although it is true that doctors are running away from a possible meeting point with technology, in this metaphor, technology has nevertheless remained firm in its position: it did not take any steps in the direction of the medical profession.

With this I absolutely do not want to say that technologies should regress to the level of training that doctors have – *knowledge must always go forward* – but it is true that artificial intelligences, in order to be adopted, need to **adapt** to the particularities of the medical field and of the medical class.

Always remembering the lessons of Hygiene and Public Health of Professor Nante, mentioned in the chapter on Medicine, one of the peculiarities of medical field is the difficulty of evaluating the good it offers: Health.

While all other professions produce goods or services that are easy to assess, even economically, the same cannot be said for Medicine.

To assess the value of most goods and services, we just need to study the **law of supply and demand**, so a simple formula is enough to calculate their price.
The same cannot be said for Health. To understand why, we need to start from its definition.

"Health is a state of complete physical, mental and social well-being and not merely the absence of disease or infirmity."
(Preamble to the **Constitution of WHO** as adopted by the International Health Conference, New York, 19 June - 22 July 1946; signed on 22 July 1946 by the representatives of 61 States (Official Records of WHO, no. 2, p. 100) and entered into force on 7 April 1948. The definition has not been amended since 1948.)

Health is therefore defined by a well-being that is:
- **Physical**
- **Mental**
- **Social**

If it is true that the former is easy to evaluate, especially with the most modern imaging technologies, the same cannot be said for mental well-being, a very controversial and debated topic, nor, so much, for the social one.

In this enormously multifaceted context, Professor Nante explained to us that health also has an extremely changeable **perceived value**.

To explain this, he gave us the following example.
Let's think that we are suffering from the most atrocious headache we can experience. Our head is pounding hard, and we are suffering the pains of hell.
How much would we be willing to pay for a medicine that will heal us instantly?
Probably, at that precise moment, we would be willing to give up all our possessions to feel good again.

Still remaining in this example, let's pretend that someone gives us this medicine, without paying for it in advance.
We instantly feel good again, and we no longer have a headache.
At this point, how much would we be willing to pay for the medicine that was given to us?
It is easy that, now, the answer is very different, and that it sounds like this: as little as possible, or even nothing.

This example, however trivial, shows how changeable the perceived value of the good that hospitals offers is, and how intricate this specific area of knowledge is.

How can one quantify a good so transient, fickle and complex?

Perhaps, through professor Nante's example, we have discovered a new meaning of the phrase: **"Health is priceless"**.

Going back to talking about the **intrinsic value** of health, setting aside what is perceived, and referring to its definition, we realize that, to the physical, moral and social aspects, others are added.

One of these, which is among the social ones, is the specific value of personal **medical data**.

While, however private, a subject may wish to share some of his or her data, if adequately remunerated, the same cannot be said for clinical data.

In the ward, I could easily ask a patient how much his phone costs, where he bought it and what use he makes of it, but, if I asked him, how I did it, if and how much he smokes and if and how much he drinks, it's very likely for him tell a **lie**.

The same can be said for the use of drugs and, above all, for everything concerning the sexual sphere.

Besides this, health very often coincides with other spheres, and this makes it a field with blurred boundaries.

There are many ethical aspects, just think of the issues concerning abortion, euthanasia, organ donation, transplants, which bring people to defend or oppose them in squares and courts all around the world.

These aspects, very often, also fall into the spiritual or religious sphere, which leads them to a much higher level of complexity.
Even here, think about the themes of abortion, euthanasia, donations, or the theme of pain, which can be conceived as divine punishment, or ritual practices such as infibulation or circumcision.

While deepening the aspect of mental well-being, Medicine includes both physical and psychological well-being.
Let's think of the inability to describe psychiatric pathologies, of which the medical world does not know the etiology, does not understand the pathogenesis and does not know what their cure could be.
Not to mention that, behind any physical trauma, there is also a psychological, often misunderstood repercussion that affects each subject differently.

There are hundreds of examples of models with scarring on their face or football players with injuries that mark their entire career.

Artificial intelligences, such as doctors, will not be faced with a given pathology as described in books, nor the classic Caucasian patient of 180 cm and 70 kg, but situations so particular as to always represent exceptions, and never rules.

For this reason, new technologies, if they want to be accepted by both doctors and patients, must be able to **understand** and satisfy the needs of both.

In the following section of this chapter, we will see how it will be possible and how, even in Siena, is already happening.

4.3 – From Industry 4.0 to Healthcare 4.0

Making a brief summary of what brought us to this point, in the previous chapter the difficulty of the medical class in adopting new technologies has been described.

We have seen how there are limits on both sides, and that there also limitations inherent to their relationship.

With these premises, in this chapter, we discussed, in the first section, the paradigms of Industry 4.0.

We have emphasized the reasons why this revolution is formally and substantially different from all the others, and has infinitely greater potential and dimensions than those of previous industrial revolutions.

In the second paragraph, instead, we described the peculiarities of the medical field, since, unlike all other sectors, it has specific characteristics that make it unique, as has been explained above all with reference to the "economic" value of health.

We have, therefore, as always, on the one hand the new technologies, which, taken together and in their context, represent Industry 4.0.
On the other hand, instead, we have the doctors, with the limits concerning their figure and their profession.

In this section we will try to understand how to reconcile such a revolutionary technology with such a particular profession, laying the foundations for what is called **Healthcare 4.0**.

It is clear that the means in the hands of those who create and develop these technologies are infinitely superior to those in the hands of the doctors.
And it is also clear that the clinical knowledge of a doctor and his experience cannot be known in their entirety by an engineer or a programmer, and therefore it cannot and should not be supplanted, at least for now, by a machine.

In the course of this troubled relationship between medicine and technology, above all between artificial intelligences and clinical practice, we reached a point where experts ceased to speak about AI, and started to discuss **AIMI**, **Artificial Improvement of Medical Intelligence**.

This is the cornerstone of Healthcare 4.0.
Machines must not replace doctors, but they must be powerful and precise tools placed in their hands.

Artificial intelligences, in fact, as happens with the iDScore, must accompany the physician in the diagnostic path and, from this new relationship, mutual benefit must be drawn.

The machines, at this stage of their development, must be thought as **categorizers** of medical knowledge.
Not only that, but they must also be objectivators and quantizers of clinical acquaintance.

If, as in the case of dermatology, once upon a time an expert dermatologist could diagnose a malignant lesion with his "naked eye", now, with the use of new technologies, he must be asked: what did you notice precisely? Why is it important in your diagnosis?

In this way, we can bring into the quantitative world what, at first, was a purely and exclusively qualitative knowledge.

This is one of the key points of my thesis: technologies, little by little, must be able to describe, define and quantify what was once considered "intuition", "stroke of genius", "clinical sense".

In this way, the quantitative world will succeed in extracting from the qualitative world a knowledge that has remained too long abstract and aleatory, due to the difficulties previously illustrated.

To do this, artificial intelligences cannot compete with doctors, but must be placed at the service of clinical practice.

One way this can be done is, for example, to convert complex AI algorithms and difficult statistical calculations into a score system.

Although it may seem trivial, it is a subterfuge with which new technologies can be adopted by doctors without them noticing, but not only: without even having them use the computer.

In the next chapter, in fact, we will see specifically how this happened and is happening with the iDScore in the Dermatology Department of the University of Siena.

Like when **Julius Caesar** conquered Gaul leaving, a little at a time, more and more Roman legionaries in the service of the Gallic tribes; even the new technologies, at first, will have to win the trust of professional workers by bowing their heads in front of them.

The iDScore, in fact, having as its facade a simple score system, as there are many, actually hides years of studies carried out at European level and an artificial intelligence that performs an enormous amount of calculations, which doctors could not do, and that they are not even required to know.

In this way, the complexity of the medical world corresponds to the power of artificial intelligences, and the inability of doctors to adopt new technologies corresponds to a simple, immediate and intuitive interface that makes them able to use them.

The humanization of machines (AI to AIMI) and the quantization of clinical practice (AIMI to AI), gestures with the same direction, but with opposite verse, if performed both, can lead to the adoption of Industry 4.0 technologies in the medical world, giving rise to Healtchare 4.0.

The next chapter, in fact, will focus on an example of AI application in the Dermatology Department of Siena: the iDScore Project, developed in the last few years and whose present thesis contributes to its updating.

"One machine can do the work of fifty ordinary men. No machine can do the work of one extraordinary man."

Elbert Green Hubbard

Chapter 5.

AI in dermatology

The fifth chapter of my thesis focuses on the development and the application of the iDScore platform, as a practical example of AIMI and Healthcare 4.0.

The iDscore is a score system that, by analyzing and rating certain anamnestic and dermoscopic features, is able to say a priori if a lesion is an atypical nevus (AN, and therefore a benign lesion which needs, at most, a follow up) or a melanoma (MM, and therefore a dangerous and lethal malignant lesion).

As the name implies, the project is represented by a score model.

The main score models currently used in the medical field will therefore be presented, highlighting the characteristics and, above all, the advantages and benefits that they can bring to clinical practice.

The iDS is also based on a neural network, whose functioning will be described after the one of the score systems, and it has been created by using a multicentric platform.

The platform, in fact, developed in Siena, in a first phase of the project was exported throughout Europe for the collection of lesions and the first valuations on the actual accuracy of the algorithm.

This was made possible through the creation of a cloud system that connected all the centers that took part in the project, sharing the images uploaded by them and their assessments, thus increasing the accuracy of the score and demonstrating its effectiveness in various and important European centers.

After that, the results of the study will be presented and, at this point, the section on the further improvement of the platform will be introduced.

During this academic year, in fact, I collected new data that allowed us to study how the accuracy of the platform could be further increased.

The study focused on the search for **new anamnestic variables** which, integrated with the already tested score, could even improve its performances.

The thesis will demonstrate that this objective has been achieved and that the accuracy of the model has been increased up to an astonishing and unmatched **91%**.

In addition, clinical experience, the effective application of the model in real time during the visits, was able to demonstrate a particular effectiveness in the recognition and management, in real time and live, of the **diagnostic error**.

This, as will be widely discussed in the last parts of the chapter, opens up a range of possibilities: if the doctor and the score reach a different diagnosis, or if the score and the histology itself reach a different diagnosis, given the extremely high accuracy of the score model, who will be right? And, moreover, how can we know it?

The chapter will end by addressing current and future perspectives; the latter will be widely resumed and deepened in the last part of this paper.

5.1 – Present and future of AI in Dermatology

The purpose of this section is to outline the state of the art concerning the adoption of artificial intelligences in the medical field, in general, and in the dermatological field, in particular.

Already in the second chapter of this script, in fact, many examples of artificial intelligences currently in use in clinical practice have been described, however, in the medical field, as it has been shown, they still represent exceptions – rather than the rule – contrary to what happens in all other areas.

The examples, in fact, fall into the definition of "*shiny machines*" of which a hospital boasts and on which many scientific and newspaper articles are written, however, as we have seen, those technologies are not the norm, and the reality is often completely different.

The reality that doctors and patients face is often the one described in the third chapter of this paper, in which doctors often fear the technologies that, as mentioned, they do not know, and tend to overlap them with the figure of bureaucracy.

Things, fortunately, are beginning to change.

To that end, we can mention **Medica**, the **World Forum for Medicine**, the most important international medical fair, to be held in November 2019 in Düsseldorf, Germany.

Below is the image of the poster.

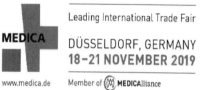
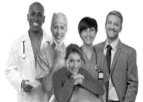

As it is widely explained on their website, whose link will be present in the sitography of the paper, being the most important medical fair in the World, it represents a forerunner for everything concerning the medical world, posing as a bridge between present and future of healthcare.

Fairs like this, or like **Arab Health**, held in January 2020 and presented below, discuss, years in advance, what, with time, will become the vanguard of clinical practice.

It is no coincidence that the main theme of both fairs is the use of artificial intelligences in the clinical practice.

So it is true that the medical community is late on the roadmap of the adoption of new technologies, but, at least, it is also true that the entire scientific community is beginning to recognize their immense value and, more importantly, even as far as medical practice is concerned, we are beginning to discuss which repercussions artificial intelligence will have.

Below is presented the Arab Health poster, "the largest gathering of healthcare and rade professionals", which shows the origin of the participants in the event.

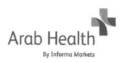

Arab Health
By Informa Markets

Who attends

Arab Health is the largest gathering of healthcare and rade professionals in the MENA regions, welcoming over 55,000 attendees from 159 countries.

Visitors by region

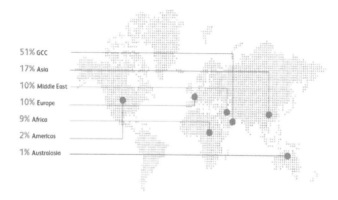

51% GCC
17% Asia
10% Middle East
10% Europe
9% Africa
2% Americas
1% Australasia

The same can be said that it is also happening in the dermatological field.

In fact, during the month of June, Dr. Tognetti took part in the **World Congress of Dermatology**, held in Milan.

Dr. Tognetti there presented the iDScore platform, based on an artificial intelligence, to the whole world; the iDS represents a meeting point between the dermatology department of Siena, directed by professor Rubegni, and the engineering world, in the figure of professor Cevenini, both founders and developers of the project.

At the event she also saw how all the dermatologists in the world are walking, often more in the intention than in practice, the road that will lead them to the adoption of artificial intelligences.

Which, as we shall see, with the iDScore, in Siena is already a reality.

The poster of the event is presented below, in which Dr. Tognetti took part to demonstrate the efficacy of the iDScore and to compare her with the rest of the world on the most important and current issues concerning dermatology.

It is no coincidence that the subtitle speaks of "**A new ERA for global Dermatology**".

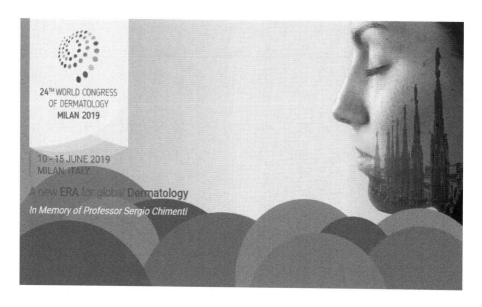

The theme of artificial intelligences, in fact, is so important that it is not only treated in all international medical and dermatological fairs, but there are specific conferences, with experts from all over the world, explicitly on this theme.

An example is that to which Professor Rubegni invited us, presented in the following image.

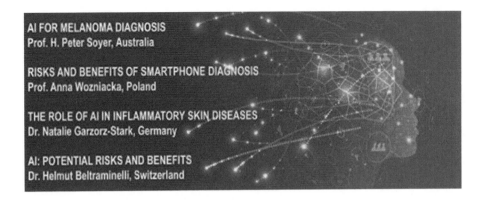

AI FOR MELANOMA DIAGNOSIS
Prof. H. Peter Soyer, Australia

RISKS AND BENEFITS OF SMARTPHONE DIAGNOSIS
Prof. Anna Wozniacka, Poland

THE ROLE OF AI IN INFLAMMATORY SKIN DISEASES
Dr. Natalie Garzorz-Stark, Germany

AI: POTENTIAL RISKS AND BENEFITS
Dr. Helmut Beltraminelli, Switzerland

It is of fundamental importance that even the medical world, even if with abundant delay, begins to address these issues.

Dermatology, in fact, being mainly based on the recognition of images, accompanied by anamnestic variables, as well as radiology, can benefit enormously from a conscious adoption of artificial intelligences.

If it is true that the medical world, little by little, is recognizing the benefits of new technologies, it is also true that this is still too little.

In the previous chapter, we saw, in fact, that doctors present gaps that are very difficult to fill; and, in the previous section, we have discovered that they are much more evident in medical practice than in all other professions.

We cannot pretend that all problems are solved simply by recognizing their existence, nor speaking about them for a few hours at a conference of a few days.

It is a starting point, though.

One more step, however, has been made by the University of Siena which, with the iDScore, presented in the next section, put into practice, as it has already been doing for some years, the technologies that the world is now beginning to speak about.

5.2 – An AI application: the iDScore Project

"The clinical diagnosis of melanoma could be challenging and dermoscopy increases the diagnostic accuracy of clinical examination. The iDScore checklist was designed as an integrated clinical-dermoscopic risk scoring system aimed to support dermatologists dealing with clinically and dermoscopically "difficult" melanocytic skin lesions suggestive for melanoma. The training and first testing set were developed with expert dermoscopists over a dataset of 435 lesions (134 early melanomas and 301 atypical nevi) with a high diagnostic accuracy (area under the ROC curve of 0.90)"
(Tognetti, Aug 29, 2019)

In the dermatological field, at present, attempts have been made to use artificial intelligences to define the malignancy of the lesions.

Through the use of the dermoscope, in fact, a tool that allows to acquire magnified and standardized images, doctors tried to make use of **image recognition** to define the diagnosis and, consequently, the prognosis of the patients.

However, over the years, it has been realized that the score models, such as the iDScore, as more accurate and extremely easier to understand and therefore to use, represent the best possible support for dermatological diagnosis, combining speed, intuitiveness, accuracy and practicality.

Scores, in Medicine, as well as checklists (as the iDS is described by Doctor Tognetti in the most recent paper about the iDScore) have always been widely used and infinitely important.

A score, in fact, is a model that assigns a scoring to each risk factor and to each symptom related to a specific pathology, these scores are then eventually multiplied by coefficients that indicate how important the characteristics associated with them are, and, in the end, a sum is made.

If the sum is above a certain cut off, it is likely that the disease is present, and further investigations or treatment are therefore advised; if the score is below the cut off, another process is followed.

Through the use of a specific score, in fact, it is possible to obtain a faster and more correct diagnosis, since it is done in a systematic, rapid, and automated way.

The score systems therefore have many advantages, in fact they are:

- Quick
- Easy to apply
- Precise
- Evidence based
- Automatic
- They reduce errors and forgetfulness of doctors

- They are, at least in part, objectivable

- They can be considered as an equal standard in all parts of the World.

The easiest score model is the one without coefficients, or, better to say, the one in which the coefficient is always equal to 1 (k = 1).

Consequently, the doctor, the patient, or any citizen, will often simply have to learn a short acronym that allows him to quickly remember all the parameters of the score.

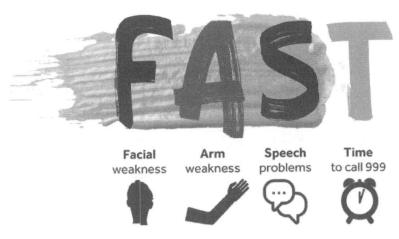

| **Facial** weakness | **Arm** weakness | **Speech** problems | **Time** to call 999 |

Learn it. Share it. You could save a life.

An example is the acronym **F.A.S.T.**, which allows to diagnose the possible presence of a stroke.

Other important examples can be the scores used to determinate whether a patient is suffering of pulmonary emobolism (PE) or not.

For those interested, the scores that I mentioned are explained and deepened in **Appendix A**, at the end of the paper, in order to better understand their functioning.

Friendly to the doctor and the patient, so that it is accepted and welcomed as a simple method that integrates perfectly into the usual clinical practice and makes it immediately and fully perceive the usefulness and effectiveness.

"Score models are ideal for the dermoscopy, where many subjective dichotomous variables with redundant information can be selected and added to binarized clinical-anamnestic variables, in order to form integer scores with high diagnostic accuracy. The individual diagnostic abilities of several experienced dermatologists can be integrated and enhanced into an instrument in performance far superior to each of them individually."

(Cevenini, 2016).

However, many of these scores have the characteristic of being static, which is a great limitation, or, rather, they are updated with a very low frequency, often following consensus.

The iDScore, instead, as we will see, while remaining equally simple to apply, is much more sophisticated and fast adapting, since it's based on an AI.

In dermatology, the biggest challenge is to distinguish melanomas (MM) from atypical nevi (AN).

Melanoma is a malignant neoplastic lesion, with a strong tendency to metastasize, and that, being practically free of signs and symptoms, has an extremely high lethality.

The atypical nevus, on the other hand, is a benign lesion, virtually harmless, but that, over time, can turn into a melanoma.

In case of melanoma, treatment is surgical. However, it is essential that the diagnosis is early, otherwise even surgery cannot improve patient survival.

In the case of the atypical nevus, instead, the treatment involves the simple follow-up. The frequency of follow-up is directly proportional to the presumed malignant potential of the lesion.

What is the problem, then?
The problem is that a melanoma and an atypical nevus are very similar, and it is therefore easy to confuse them.

However, since the lethality of melanoma is very high, in case of doubt, the lesion is removed.

This leads to an incredible number of false positives (FP) and a disproportionate increase in public spending in order to remove them.

Also, in dermatology many scores and checklists have been introduced to facilitate the diagnosis of melanoma.

Some examples include:

- Pattern analysis,
- Seven Point checklist,
- The ABCD rule (A: Asymmetry, B: Borders, C: Color, D: Diameter), shown in the following image.

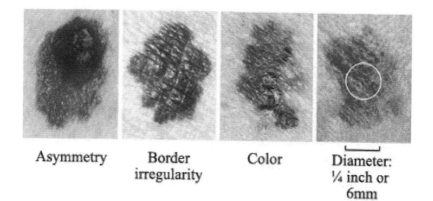

Asymmetry   Border   Color   Diameter:
             irregularity   ¼ inch or
                                   6mm

However, the accuracy of these models is still very low, and this led to the development of the iDScore platform by Professor Cevenini et al.

The iDS integrates anamnestic variables and dermoscopic criteria and, as we will understand, has an accuracy much higher than that of the models previously presented.

The research in which I have been involved is focused on further improving the accuracy of the AI-based algorithm.

5.3 – Teledermatology web platform in cloud computing

This section explains how the iDScore platform has been designed.

The platform, as said, integrating clinical-anamnestic and dermoscopic variables, is used in the assessment of malignancy risk.

To carry out this study, **435** standardized dermoscopic images of clinically atypical melanocytic skin lesions (MSL) removed in suspected malignancy were selected, of which:

- **134** (31%) were early melanomas (EM), and
- **301** (69%) were atypical nevi (AN).

For each injury, the following clinical variables have been collected:

Regarding the patient:
- **Age** (years),
- **Sex** (M/F).

As for the lesion:
- **Dimension** (mm),
- **Site of the lesion** (group A, "upper extremities": head, neck, arms and hands; group B, "lower extremities": thighs, legs, legs, ankles and back of the foot; group C, "upper trunk": shoulders, back and chest; group D: "lower trunk").

Afterwards, three experts (unaware of both the histological diagnosis and the clinical-anamnestic characteristics) evaluated the presence or absence of 12 dermoscopic structures by compiling a predefined evaluation form – reported in the table – for a total of 1305 dermoscopic evaluations (Tognetti, Cevenini et al., 2018).

Dermoscopic variables	Abbreviation	Definition
1. Atypical network	AN	Irregularly meshed pigmented network irregularly distributed through the lesion
2. Irregular dots and globules	IDG	Sharply circumscribed, round to oval, rown to black structures of variously sized and irregular distribution
3. Irregular streaks	IS	Peripheral brownish to black lines/pseudopods of variable thickness and length, not combined with pigment network lines
4. Irregular pigmented blotches	IPB	Brown to black irregularly pigmented area circumscribed that precludes recognition of subtler dermoscopic structures
5. Blue with veil BWV <30% BWV >30%	BWV	Irregular, superficial veil consisting of a confluent, white-blue to whitish-blue pigmentation
6. Blue-grey globules	BGG	Oval structures of blue to bluish appearance
7. Blue-grey peppering	BGP	Fine blue/grey/blue-grey pepper-like structures
8. White scar-like areas	WSA	White areas with scar-like appearance
9. Shiny white streaks	SWS	Linear structures with shiny white colour
10. Hypopigmented areas	HA	Defined interruption of the pigmented network/dermoscopic structures, resulting in structureless areas within a structured area
11. Atypical vascular pattern	AVP	The presence of two or more of the following type of vessel: hairpin, dotted, linear, irregular, corkscrew, polymorphic vessels
12. Pink areas	PA	Pink/pinkish shade/milky-red areas that interfere with the recognition of the other dermoscopic structures

The interobserver agreement of the dermoscopic evaluations was calculated from Cohen's Kappa Coefficient for each pair of examiners.

The average of the Kappa value and its standard deviation were used to assess the concordance level of each dermoscopic variable and the general diagnosis by dermatologists by using the Altman scale as the reference scale.

Subsequently, the experts were asked to give an **intuitive diagnosis** on the dermoscopic images in order to create an integrated database so that for each image there were three subjective dermoscopic assessments and objective clinical-anamnestic data.

For each lesion, 16 predictive variables were considered, that were:

- 12 dermoscopic variables,
- 2 clinical variables (maximum diameter and location of the lesion)
- 2 anamnestic variables (age and sex).

Sex was coded as M/F, a value from 1 to 4 was given for the four body areas previously described, while quantitative variables such as age and diameter were binarized by taking quartiles (Q1, Q2, Q3) corresponding to 5 mm, 7 mm and 10 mm for the diameter, and 30 years, 40 years and 60 years for the age.

Each binary predictor was coded 0/1 according to the clinical significance of the low/high risk of malignancy.

The iDScore itself was then developed in three phases:

- First of all, a gradual logistic regression approach was applied in order to select the subset of significant interdependent dermoscopic variables with the highest discriminating power for malignancy (the number of dermoscopic features selected in each lesion was expressed as "dermatoscopic sum", Dsum).

- Subsequently, the Dsum variable and the four clinical anamnestic variables were introduced in another logistic classifier, to be evaluated through their gradual entry into the logistic model.
 Thus, the scoring system was obtained by rounding the regression coefficients of the previous logistic classifier to their nearest integer values, and then added together to obtain the final score S.
 The threshold level St of the score was established in a way that the lesions with S > St were classified as malignant, with the highest possible level of sensitivity (SE.) and the lowest possible level of specificity (SP.).

- The "leave one out" cross validation method was then used to obtain a high level of generalization, in which all cases were used both for the training phase and for the testing phase.

The area under the ROC curve (AUC) of the LOO was considered as a performance criterion at every step in selecting the significative characteristics.

Therefore, the procedure was interrupted in step 9, when the AUC reached the maximum value, to avoid overfitting.

Furthermore, the 95% CI for the AUC was estimated, and the full score model was designed using **Matlab** software and the 10th **SPSS** version.

In conclusion, the interdependent significant variables selected by the classifier were:

- 7 dermoscopic characteristics (atypical network, AN; irregular streaks, IS; irregular dots and globules, IDG; blu-white veil, BWV; blue-gray peppering, BGP; white scar-like areas, WSA; shiny white streaks, SWS)
- 3 age ranges (30-40 years, 41-60 years and >60 years),
- 2 categories of diameters (6-10 mm and >11 mm),
- 3 body areas (A, B and C).

The following is the iD Score checklist:

Variables	Assessment	Coefficients
Seven dermoscopic structures (Dsum)	AN present	1
	IS present	1
	IDG present	1
	BWV present	1
	BGP present	1
	WSA present	1
	SWS present	1
Three lesion sites	Upper extremities – *chronically photoexposed*: head-neck/arms/hands	2
	Lower extremities – *frequently photoexposed*: thighs/legs/ankles/back of the feet	2
	Upper trunk – *seldom photoexposed*: shoulders/back/chest/breast	1
Two maximum diameter categories	6–10 mm	3
	≥11 mm	4
Three age groups	30–40 years	1
	41–60 years	2
	≥61 years	3
Dsum partial score + clinical-personal partial score =		Total score (S)

Subsequently, the same database employed for the training phase was then used also in the testing phase to diagnose the various lesion, using the checklist created.

Using all the values of S (from 0 to 16) for the different thresholds (St), different values of SP and SE were obtained. Said values allowed to construct the ROC curve that represented the performance of the iDScore model.

In particular, a ROC curve calculated with a 95% CI (0.887-0.918) provided an AUC of 0.993; the best level of accuracy is with St ≥ 6, with SE = 94.8% and SP = 68%.

Using only the Pattern analysis, on the other hand, a level of SE = 61.7% and SP = 76.9% were reached. Therefore, by making use of the iDScore checklist, the experts could increase their diagnostic capacity.

The scale of S criticality values could be defined as follows:

- from **0** to **5**: the lesions can be considered uncritical, so there is no risk of malignancy,
- from **6** to **9**: average criticality,
- from **10** to **16**: high criticality.

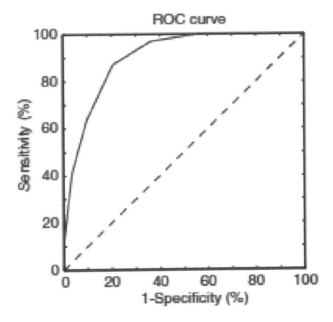

Based on what has been shown, the scoring systems are a class of engaging and intuitive clinical predictive models since the score can be calculated without using any data processing system, as we will see in the context of my clinical experience, presented in the upcoming sections.

The scores combine simplicity and extreme ease of use and provide good diagnostic accuracy, especially when a large number of predictive variables are available.

Scoring models are ideal for dermoscopy, where many subjective dichotomous variables with redundant information can be selected and added to the clinical-anamnestic binarized variables in order to form whole scores with high diagnostic precision.

Furthermore, the individual diagnostic abilities of several experienced dermatologists can be integrated and improved into an instrument with performances far superior to each of them individually.

Finally, these models make it possible to interpret the conditions of malignancy more concisely, focusing on a smaller number of risk factors and reducing the dermatoscopic analysis time.

Cloud

The creation of a cloud platform dedicated to teledermoscopy (TWP) was fundamental within the EADV project "European web platform for the development of a Scoring Classifier for Early Melanoma detection".

The cloud platform made it possible to achieve important goals:

- Create an integrated database of high quality dermoscopic images from various European centers

- Evaluate the diagnostic performance of the iDScore method by comparing it with the performances obtainable both with an "intuitive" diagnosis and with two other assessment tools, the Seven Point Check list and the ABCD rule, among the most common methods of support for diagnosis used in clinical dermatology.

The web platform, designed to achieve these two objectives, is a versatile platform that is accessible from different types of devices, such as PCs, smartphones and tablets, is based on secure and highly optimized communication systems, and is characterized by two main parts:

- The first part (accessible to the URL: eadv-idscore.dbm.unisi.it) was the "project" website through which the image archive was created, and the recruitment activities of the testing phase took place.
It is accessible by the various subjects involved in the construction of the archive, in particular by **dermatologists** (responsible for the collection of the images and for the recruitment to the testing procedures in the clinical centers involved) and by the **engineers** - responsible for quality control and post-image processing.

- The second part (accessible to the URL: idscore.dbm.unisi.it) was instead the "testing session website", accessible to all participants recruited for the testing phase.

A total of 8 **European centers** took part in the iDScore Project (Siena, St. Etienne, Nice, Naples, Barcelona, Reggio Emilia and Thessaloniki) and, for each center, a researcher was designated as responsible for the collection of a minimum of 70 up to a maximum of 100 images of clinically atypical melanocytic skin lesions that have already been excised due to suspicion of malignancy.

The criteria for selecting the images were:

- image/case of good quality,
- 17X-20X magnification range,
- ≥1 Mpx, ≥150 DPI,
- contact polarized dermatoscopy,
- JPEG format,
- availability of 5 clinical/anamnestic data, including body area localization, maximum diameter (mm), age (years) and patient sex (M/F), plus the histological diagnosis AN/EA (Atypical nevus/Early melanoma).

A 9-month period was dedicated to this database creation phase and, by the time of site closure, 1000 images were collected, 21 of which were discarded because they did not meet the quality standards, while 979 constituted the final database.

Subsequently, each researcher responsible for the site was asked to recruit at least 20 participants with different levels of competence in dermatoscopy:

- level 1: <1 year of experience;
- level 2: 1-4 years of experience;
- level 3: 5-8 years of experience;
- level 4: ≥9 years of experience.

A standardized email was sent to each participant containing a personal registration URL, automatically generated by the invitation procedure.

The users of the web platform were enabled to access them from different devices and, on first access, information on the entire project was provided to all the participants.

Once the registration and participation policies were accepted, the participant was provided with an identification code (a personal token) for the login and, after authenticating, the user had to fill out a profiling form.

During this phase, the affiliate link was registered between each participant and the researcher from whom he was recruited, in order to ensure that the images that would have been submitted to him did not come from the same center where he worked, thus allowing a completely blind examination.

All the participants, a total of 111 between doctors and doctoral students of different levels of experience, once registered through the personal token, were enabled to enter the testing session of the platform.

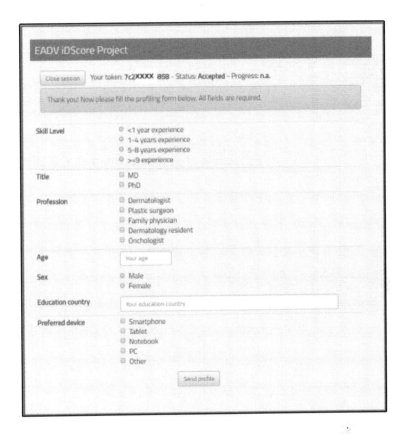

The testing session could be suspended and restarted without any restriction and performed with any device; the only limitation was that all participants were required to complete the test within 120 days of starting it.

Each participant was subjected to the evaluation of a dataset of 30 randomly selected cases from the integrated dermoscopic database software, calibrated so as to provide a 4:1 ratio between each of the AN and EM cases, generated in this way in order to simulate the actual frequency with which lesions occur in clinical practice.

To improve its visualization, each image could have been enlarged within the display available area of the browser window, and, to each image of the dataset, four icons (corresponding to four panels) were associated.

PANEL	CONTENT	REQUEST
Panel I	Dermoscopic and clinical image Patient and injury data	Select an "intuitive diagnosis" between EM and MM and decide the management mode between follow-up, no follow-up, no preventive excision.
Panel II	Dermoscopic image and iDScore calculation grid	Evaluate using iDScore checklis

Panel III	Dermoscopic and clinical image	Evaluate the 4 criteria, asymmetry, borders, colors and dermoscopic structures, according to the ABCD rules scoring system
Panel IV	Dermoscopic and clinical image	Evaluate through the 7-point checklist

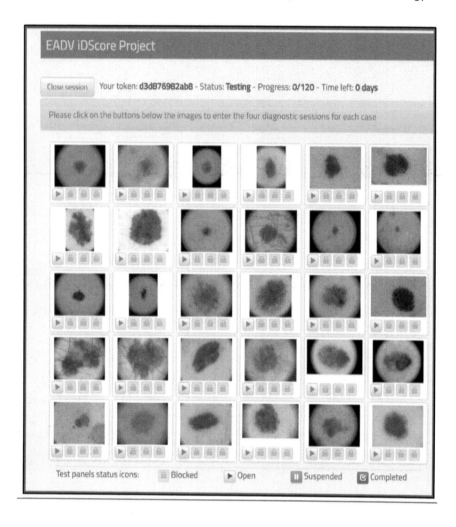

After completing the test session, the participants were able to access the final report page.

- In the first screen, the histological diagnosis of all cases evaluated was revealed to users, and the results of panel 1 evaluations were indicated on each dermoscopic image as true positive (TP), true negative (TN), false positive (FP) and false negative (FN), according to the correct/wrong answers.

- On the second page, instead, the diagnostic performances obtained with the 4 different methods have been reported, in terms of area under the ROC curve (AUC), their accuracy (ACC), sensitivity (SE) and specificity (SP), value positive predictive (PPV) and negative predictive value (NPV), taking as a score threshold ≥7 for the iDScore test, ≥5.45 for the ABCD test and ≥3 for the Seven Point checklist (Tognetti, Cevenini et al., 2018).

Close session Your token: 8e087c4c6588 - Status: **Done** - Progress: **120/120** - Time left: **n.a.**

Click the button below to return to the session panel

Testing session results

	Pattern analysis	iDScore	ABCD Rule	7-Point Checklist
AUC	0.73	0.93	0.87	0.89
SP	0.65	0.35	0.85	0.20
SE	0.80	1.00	0.80	1.00
ACC	0.70	0.57	0.83	0.47
PPV	0.53	0.43	0.73	0.38
NPV	0.87	1.00	0.89	1.00

AUC Specificity Sensitivity Accuracy Positive Predictive Value Negative Predictive Value

Pattern analysis

iDScore

ABCD Rule

7-Point Checklist

5.4 – iDScore project results

As said, a total of 979 injuries were collected, assessed by 111 participants, for a total of 3330 assessments from 8 European centers (Siena: 41%, Barcelona: 6%, Thessaloniki: 2%, Modena: 12%, Reggio Emilia: 1% , Nice: 7%, Naples: 26%, St. Etienne: 1%).

The evaluations were carried out by different types of devices, which see the prevalent use of PC (42%) and smarthpone (16%).

To analyze user performance with the various evaluation methods, the ROC curve and the average area under the ROC curve (AUC) were calculated:

- for the iDScore it was **0.776** [CI: 95%, 0.760-0.792],
- for the 7 Point checklist it was 0.698 [CI: 95%, 0.670-0.707],
- for ABCD rule it was 0.698 [CI: 95%, 0.979-0.716],

- for intuitive diagnosis it was 0.674 [CI: 95%, 0.655-0.693].

(Tognetti, Aug 29, 2019).

The potential contribution that the web platform and the iDScore are able to offer in educational terms has already been demonstrated through the observable results in the AUC differentiated for the four levels of experience of those who performed the test using the four rating methods.

As can be seen from the graph, the iDScore was the method by which participants, regardless of their skill level, achieved the best performance.

In particular, choosing a threshold ≥7 for the iDScore, values **SE = 86%** and **SP = 52%** were reached, while with score thresholds ≥8 and ≥6, the levels that would have been obtained would be, respectively: SE = 76% and SP = 66%, and SE = 92% and SP = 36%.

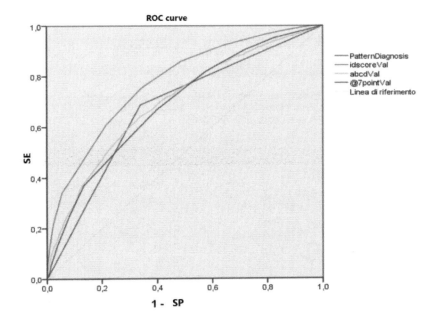

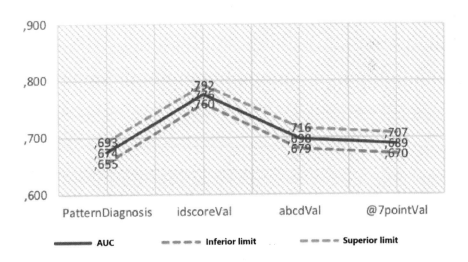

In fact, all groups have improved their performance from the intuitive diagnosis to that assisted by the iDScore.

In particular, level 1 dermatologists (dermatologicals with the lowest level of experience) managed to improve their performance by an extraordinary **20%**.

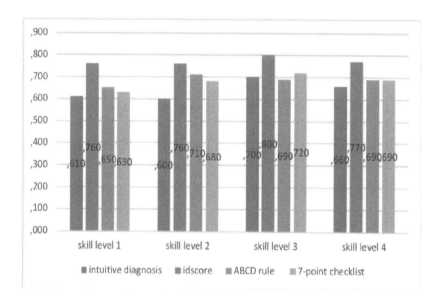

The use of a TWP platform and the introduction of diagnostic tools such as the iDScore, able to improve the accuracy of the diagnosis, can have a strong relevance both on the expectation and on the quality of life of the individual, and on the cost reduction for health.

In this context, the main factors that determine a strong cost reduction are:

- The detection of melanoma at an earlier stage, with a consequent reduction in the costs related to treatment, and
- The reduction of excisions for suspicious lesions, which would impact on total health costs, as they are strongly linked to the number of false positives (FP) obtained during the diagnostic process.

An annual estimate of costs related to excisions varies according to the type of treatment:

- from $151 in the case of benign injury,
- to $2974 for the broader excisions,
- up to $125239 for the treatment of metastatic melanoma of stage III and IV.
  (G.Watts et al 2016).

In general, the treatment of patients diagnosed with malignant melanoma guarantees an average life expectancy of around 11.5 months, with an average cost of $30000, or about $2668 per month per patient (Mc Marron et al.2015).

The costs have been calculated without taking into account the fact that, in the next few years, in addition to the classical chemotherapic treatment, with which metastatic melanoma is now generally treated, **immunotherapy treatments** will be increasingly widespread, which will show a significant improvement in the increase in life expectancy.

As a result of their incredible clinical benefit, these new drugs are sold at extremely high prices - far superior to those of current chemotherapy.

For this reason, investments in research must go hand in hand with those linked to prevention and improvement in the accuracy of diagnoses.

The estimated costs that will have to be addressed in the future by the health service will be around €269682 per patient, of which €215150 are related to immunity therapy and only €44165 will be spent for hospitalization (M.Kandel et al., 2018).

5.5 – My contribution to iDScore clinical testing and improvement

In September 2018 I asked for a meeting to one of the fathers of the iDScore project, Professor Cevenini, who gave me the opportunity to take part in the development and **improvement** of the platform, attending the Dermatology Department of Siena, directed by professor Rubegni.

My field of research was divided into two parts:

- In the first one I should have collected the anamnestic data of patients whose lesions had already been removed, to evaluate the effectiveness of the iDScore, and to look for other characteristics that could improve its already high accuracy;

- While, in the second, I applied the iDScore practically and physically in the department, to demonstrate its immediacy, intuitiveness and speed of application.

In the first part of my study I therefore contacted 100 patients. 50 of these had had a melanoma (MM) removed, while an atypical nevus (AN) had been removed from the other 50.

All the lesions, already removed, were provided with histological diagnoses and dermoscopic images that met the platform validity criteria.

I then collected the two data related to the patient, age and sex, and the two data related to the lesion, i.e. diameter and area of the body in which it is located.

After that, I had each lesion analyzed by three expert dermatologists, that weren't aware of the histological diagnosis nor of the clinical characteristics of the patient.

One of these three experts was Professor Rubegni, chief of Dermatology Department of Siena, who took personally part in the study.

At this point, when at least two dermatologists out of three decreed that a lesion had a given dermoscopic characteristic of those of the iDScore (atypical network, irregular streaks, blue white veil, blue grey peppering, white scar-like areas, shiny white streaks and irregular dots and globules), this feature was marked as present.

On the contrary, if two or more dermatologists said that the characteristic was absent, a zero (= absence) was marked on the associated box.

This step was carried out to minimize possible errors and to have greater concordance.

Then, for each individual lesion, the iDScore was calculated, which proved to have an incredible **91% accuracy**.

And this is the first result of the study, confirming the accuracy of Siena's score to be higher than the one of all the others, as already established in the previous section.

Now it was time to try to even increase the iDS' accuracy.

The aim of this part of the research was to **identify new variables** that could improve the accuracy of the score system.

We therefore considered the following variables:

- Familiarity for melanoma, both in first-degree and second-degree relatives. Familiarity, in fact, is one of the main cancer risk factors,
- Familiarity for non melanous skin cancer (NMSC),
- The presence of phenomelanin in the patient, i.e. if the patient has red hair or freckles,
- The phototype,
- If the patient was blond,

- If the patient had clear eyes (green, light blue or blue),
- The number of nevi on the right arm (the cut-off was 11),
- If the patient had a positive medical history for sunburn. So, if he had a memory of being sunburned when he was less than 14 years old,
- If the patient smokes,
- If the patient, on average, drinks more or less than 2 glasses of red wine a day.

Statistical analysis based on the data that I collected has shown that the **phototype**, including also the characteristic **"blond hair"**, is the only one able to improve the performance of the score.

This is also perfectly in line with the most recent studies on melanoma risk factors (M.Olsen, March 2019) and has therefore the potential to **improve the model** and thus to introduce new knowledge.

Further research on a wider population will be conducted in order to have a greater statistical significance before considering adding this new parameter to the score.

Artificial Intelligence in the management and recognition of diagnostic error

However, during this study, there have been two important events that deserve special attention.

Once the data analysis was done, it was reported that two injuries, despite having a particularly low iDScore (4 and 5, respectively) had been diagnosed as melanomas.

Professor Cevenini, therefore, as a platform developer, pointed out to us the peculiarity highlighted by the algorithm and asked us to re-check these lesions in order to verify the correctness of the diagnosis.

- The first lesion, the one with iDScore = 4, in fact, due to a transcription error, was marked as a melanoma (MM), when, in reality, it was an atypical nevus (AN).

  The platform, therefore, was able to **highlight a human error** and to indicate it precisely, so that the data relating to the injury were reviewed.

- The second lesion, the one with iDScore = 5, represents an even more particular and interesting case.

  This time, in fact, a transcription error was not reported, but something much more important happened.

  All the lesion data were checked and, once they were found to be all correct, the histological diagnosis was reviewed.

The histological diagnosis reported that the one removed was a borderline lesion, which the specific anatomopathologist in question had decided to define as a melanoma.

However, the lesion, subjected to a new examination by Professor Rubegni and Dr. Tognetti, both founders and members of the iDScore Project, turned out to be "a head or cross injury", since it could be defined, with equal fairness, both as an early melanoma (EM) and an atypical nevus (AN).

At this point, it is also important to note that the value of 5 is the highest value of the low risk category of the iDS: therefore, the score, too, had underlined how much the lesion was **on the border between benignity and malignancy**.

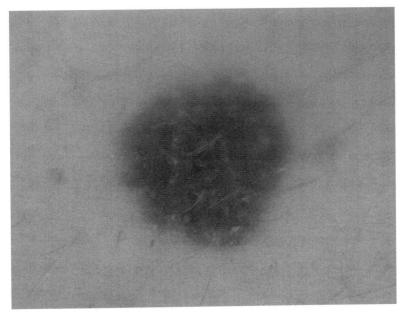

The borderline lesion with iDS=5

The results of this part of the study are three, and they are very important:

1. The iDScore confirmed that it has a very high accuracy, even **91%** in this study, confirming itself above all the other score models used in dermatology.

   Its use, even simply for this aspect, should be taken into consideration, because it has proved to be an easy, fast and above all accurate model, and, with the addition of an extra variable (the phototype, including hair color) it will be even more so.

195

2. **Correcting a human error**, he demonstrated, once more, the superiority of artificial intelligences over human ones in the performance of specific tasks.

   This is a very important point, in fact, the clinician has been invited to recheck the correctness of his diagnosis and this can avoid both false positives (FP), which entail enormous expenses for the State, and false negatives (FN), which increase the lethality (and in turn the costs) of the disease, condemning patients to death.

   Therefore, a score model, based on an artificial intelligence, however simple, being more efficient than men, is able to help them, correcting them, and then putting them and their diagnosis into discussion.

   This is an enormous benefit, given that, from a single mistake, both the artificial intelligence and the doctor can learn, and, of this correction, it can benefit both the individual patient and, indirectly, the entire Health System.

3. The model, although easy to apply, is **extremely flexible** and has all the features that allow it to represent the many facets of reality.

   As in the case of the borderline lesion with iDScore=5; such a score, indeed, perfectly represented the condition of the lesion.

A score like this, in the ward, can lead the doctor to seek the opinion of another expert, thus reducing the risk of error.

At this point, a profound reflection arises: if the score and histology give two different diagnoses, which of the two is the right one?

Considering also the times and the costs of both of them, which of the two must be taken into consideration?

Regarding this last point, however, it is necessary to make a further clarification.

Often, during the course of our studies, we are told that in medicine it is not all black or white.

A benign lesion, as a matter of fact, following a path that goes from anaplasia to dysplasia, during its evolution, is often found to be in a "**gray area**" in which it can be defined as benign by some dermatologists, or malignant by others.

It is important, therefore, that the score is able to present this condition, which it did excellently, **stimulating clinical reasoning**, but leaving the final decision to the doctor.

This is a necessary condition for getting to the Artificial Improvement of Medical Intelligence, fundamental characteristic of Healthcare 4.0.

What can be complained, however, could be that, although iDS is fast and has a very high accuracy, it cannot be easy to apply in everyday clinical practice.

My experience in the department, however, has shown the opposite.

In the first days on the ward, while the doctor was visiting the patient, with pen and paper, I easily and quickly calculated the score.

Within a few days, then, without realizing it, I had learned by heart the scores of the iDS and then managed to calculate it in real time, thus being able to tell the doctor the result of my calculation while still inserting the data into the computer.

PARAMETER		PARTIAL SCORE (only if the parameter is present)
AGE	30 - 40 years	1
	41- 60 years	2
	> 61 years	3
DIAMETER	6-10 mm	3
	≥11 mm	4
3 BODY AREAS	CHRONICALLY PHOTOEXPOSED AREAS upper extremities	2
	FREQUENTLY PHOTOEXPOSED AREAS lower extremites	2
	OCCASIONALLY PHOTOEXPOSED AREAS superior trunk	1
7 dermoscopic pattern	Atypical Network - AN	1
	Irregular Streaks - IS	1
	Blue White Veil - BWV	1
	Blue Grey Peppering - BGP	1
	White Scar-like Areas - WSA	1
	Shiny White Streaks - SWS	1
	Irregular Dots and Globules - IDG	1
TOTAL SCORE		

The form I filled in the department

As in the case of the first part of the study, even in this circumstance I was able to say that some injuries, considered of low risk by the doctors, actually had a high score on the iDS, or vice versa.

At this point, the doctors called Professor Rubegni to decide what to do with the lesion under examination.

Many times, as in the case of the lesion with iDS = 4 of the previous section, the machine corrected the expert, forcing him to review his diagnosis.

Also, in this case, beyond the considerations on health care costs and health system benefits, it is important to remember that both the patient and the doctor, as well as the algorithm, have benefited from the use of the IT platform:

- The patient is more likely to have a correct diagnosis,
- The doctor has the opportunity to learn from his mistakes and, secondly, can have greater legal protection
- The algorithm is **improved for each new patient**, continually increasing its accuracy: the more patients there are, the more accurate the score will be.

At this point, what are the reasons to fear or not to use the iDScore? Its use is a win-win situation for all parties involved. Which will it be its future, then?

Returning to the more general topic of Artificial Intelligence, in fact, many conferences are being held, such as the one that Professor Rubegni invited us to (and shown in the image below) or Medica, that introduce a lot of dermatologists and numerous doctors to the topic of artificial intelligences.

Is it enough, though?

In my humble opinion, knowledge comes from the admission of one's ignorance.

It is easy, even for a doctor, to bask in his presumed omniscience, without ever confronting anything or anyone, above all an Artificial Intelligence, but the aim of a man of science should be to pursue knowledge and, to do this, everything must necessarily be questioned.

"Si enim fallor sum"
Augustine of Hippo

Going back to the previous question – "Is it enough, though?" – in the next section we will discuss which the next steps of the iDScore and its adoption will be.

5.6 – Future developments

In this brief section, we will discuss the possible next steps in the development and in the adoption of the iDScore.

It is important, in fact, for artificial intelligences, not to remain abstract or distant, but to become used on a daily basis even in healthcare, and it is also fundamental to continuously enhance the efficiency of the algorithms.

It is true that the 91% in accuracy of the iDS is an extremely high value, but it is also true that it can be further improved by the introduction of **new variables**.

On the other hand, there are also practical actions that hospitals can do to encourage, or even force, the adoption of new technologies.

As regards the first point, namely the improvement of the score itself, it is appropriate to make a specification.

It is correct to say that the introduction of a new value can increase the effectiveness of the model, but it is also true that, by introducing a new term in an already very complicated equation, we could weigh down the calculations, without necessarily benefiting from it.

Indeed, my study has shown that by introducing a new variable (the phototype, which also includes hair color) we can improve the performance of the algorithm, but it is a fact that trying to improve such an efficient model is very risky, and it cannot be done lightly.

For this reason, the iDScore team will carry out new and much **broader studies**, both on new injuries and on lesions that are already present on the platform, to assess with absolute certainty the actual need to introduce this new term in particular, and every other variable in general.

It is as if mine had been a pilot study, aimed at indicating the direction of future research for the **iDScore 2020**.

In fact, for the model to remain as practical and intuitive as it is now, it is important that no variables are added without having the absolute certainty of their statistical significance and practical utility.

In this field too, as in all other areas of Medicine, it is important to make an accurate analysis of the cost-benefit ratio, and all conclusions must be based on solid scientific basis.

Changing topic, and discussing the adoption of the model, one could think of incorporating it into software already on the market in the dermatological field, or, rather, of creating a

mobile application or a **computer program**, or even a **device** that favors the use of this technology through telemedicine.

At programming level, in fact, it is easy to implement to the medical history digital page a simple form, such as the one I filled-in in the clinic, that allows doctors to compile the iDScore checklist in real time.
This possibility, indeed, is frequently discussed by the iDScore Team.

The advantages, beyond the economic ones deriving from a possible commercialization of a smartphone application or a PC program, would concern the doctor, who could benefit from the opinion of an artificial intelligence whose accuracy is close to that of histological analysis; the patient, whose health would profit from increased diagnostic accuracy; the Healthcare System, which would see a decrease in expenses due to fewer false positives and false negatives; and, in this case, above all, the score.

One of the main strengths of artificial intelligences, in fact, is the ability to draw conclusions from a huge amount of data: a greater adoption of the iDScore also by students – as in my case – postgraduates and specialists, for example through the marketing of an application or if its checklist was implemented in the hospital computer forms for clinical history, would lead to the collection of a disproportionate amount of data, which would exponentially increase the accuracy of the model and advise its possible updating.

However, for now, we are only discussing the immediate future of artificial intelligences, and only in the dermatological field, and this is qualificatory.

It is difficult for the reader, by limiting the discussion to the topics that have been exposed so far, even in the first chapters, to understand what the true potentials of artificial intelligences are.
For now, in fact, AIs seem nothing more than automated statistics or digital secretaries, but this is absolutely not the case.
It is no coincidence that, according to many experts, the danger that AI poses is potentially far greater than that of **nuclear weapons**.

In order to be able to understand the repercussions that they may also have in the clinical world, we must therefore understand the general rules governing these technologies and we must evaluate a future far more distant than the immediate one.

What awaits us, then, in the future?

"Does God exist? Well I would say, not yet."
Raymond Kurzweil

Chapter 6.

What we expect in the coming years

In this last chapter of the script, the future perspectives of the use of artificial intelligences will be presented, both in the medical field, in the first sections, and, above all, in a more general context.

Although this is a thesis concerning medicine, it is important to know in depth the incredible potential of these new technologies, so as to be able to understand their developments also in clinical practice.

The topics covered in this chapter, especially in the last section, in fact, have little to do with healthcare, but we must remember that Medicine is inserted in a much wider framework and that, as we have seen, many of its inferences fall into extremely different contexts, e.g.: ethical, moral, social, religious, legal, political and philosophical, just to name a few; on all of them, the enormous revolutionary effects of artificial intelligences will be exercised.

To be honest, however, this is not the reason why I decided to discuss these controversial topics - many of them, in fact, are on the verge of science fiction - but it is because, I am convinced that, like the caterpillars on Professor Nante's leaf, many doctors have a myopic and narrow conception of Medicine; in my opinion, in fact, they live in a golden bubble that isolates them (and consequently Medicine) from the rest of the world and from the rest of the professions, but it is not wise to think that, faced with the **existential risk** that AI may pose, doctors can continue to focus only on their occupation, like horses with the arrogance-made blinders of those who believe that their profession is not only the most important of all, but also the only one that really matters.

The chapter will be divided into 3 sections:

- In the first one, the future closest to us, that of the next ten years and that we are already beginning to see, will be presented.

  In these years, in fact, artificial intelligences will behave exactly like all other new technologies throughout history, probably leading to the creation of new jobs and significant economic growth.

The same should also apply to the medical field.

- In the second part, instead, something very different will happen.

In 2029, in fact, exactly 10 years from now, a machine, according to Raymond Kurzweil and many other experts, including Elon Musk, will pass the **Turing test**, and his intelligence will therefore be comparable to that of a human being, and, from that moment, following the **Law of Accelerating Returns**, its intelligence will only increase exponentially.

This scenario will inevitably lead to massive unemployment and to the radical remodeling of society, which will have to pay people who can no longer work.

- In the third part, always clinging to Kurzweil's theories, we will find ourselves facing an unpredictable future even for the greatest experts, that will lead us to the an event that takes the name of **Technological Singularity**, and which leaves room for such strange as well as terrifying theories, like the one concerning **Roko's Basilisk**, presented in the last one.

In fact, if a machine of unlimited intelligence and knowledge is created, what will it be, if not a God?

The conclusions will concern the position that the medical class and the whole humanity will have to take, beginning with being at least aware of the existence of these possible scenarios.

6.1 - Within 10 years

The period spanning the next 10 years is what many authors, like those mentioned in the third chapter, expect to last forever.

In fact, in these years, artificial intelligences, as well as iDScore itself, will be diagnostic support tools that will accompany the doctor and the patient along the clinical path, providing more means for the first and greater power per second.

Artificial intelligences, as happens in China, can be used to carry out mass screening for specific pathologies, especially those concerning imaging methods. In China, in fact, they are used for lung cancer screening.

Even in the dermatological field, through cloud systems and teledermatology, as shown in the previous chapter, a similar use to the Chinese's can be made.

This, at first, will be of great help to the doctors, making them save a lot of time.

The immediate future, in my opinion, is that presented by the author of the book mentioned in the third chapter: AIs, little more than digital secretaries, will carry out all the automatic and repetitive tasks, so that the doctor can have more time to spend with his patients.

Bill Gates himself, in a broader context and in a more distant future, is convinced that not only doctors, but all human beings, must spend their free time dedicating it to the care of the elderly, the sick and the people dear to them.

Paradoxically, therefore, contrary to what Argenziano and Lallas maintain, machines will free men from the bureaucracy and from the use that they currently make of computers, leaving them more free time for "human interactions".

The conferences that are being held across the World, such as the one Professor Rubegni invited us to or Medica itself, point exactly in this direction.

However important this is, as said, in my opinion, it is still too little.

In my opinion, the reform that will allow us to accept these changes will have to start from elementary schools, with computer lessons that will allow children to learn how to code from an early age, thus learning to use the various programs and computer systems to their advantage and getting in contact for the first time with the quantitative world that is getting more and more important in every field of knowledge.

Let's look at the examples of Elon Musk, Mark Zuckerberg and Bill Gates: all of them learned to program from an early age, and this, combined with their brilliant mind, led them to be where they are.

I think, instead, of my classmates: none of them knows how to code, I myself learned to code a few years ago, from an online course, and many do not know how to use a computer, except to go on Facebook, and have no idea what an Artificial Intelligence is.

How can we expect, tomorrow, the new medical class to be able to respond to the enormous changes that will disrupt their profession?

Courses and conferences are a great starting point, but this is still not enough.

Even because, in the following years, the changes that society will have to face will be infinitely greater than todays.

In conclusion, even outside of the medical field, for now, the economist Gordon seems to be right, as evidenced by the various studies reported in the first chapter of the script.

But the World is changing much faster than some economists expect.

"I'm not scared of a computer passing the Turing test... I'm terrified of one that intentionally fails it."

6.2 – Within 20 years

Alan Mathison Turing (23 June 1912 – 7 June 1954) was a British mathematician, computer scientist, logician, cryptanalyst, philosopher and theoretical biologist that is widely considered to be the father of theoretical computer science and artificial intelligence and that played a central role in defeating the Nazis during Second World War (Copeland, 18 June 2012).

In his 1950 paper, *"Computing Machinery and Intelligence"*, while working at the University of Manchester, Alan Turing introduced its famous test.
It opens with the words:

"I propose to consider the question, 'Can machines think?'"

But, because "thinking" is difficult to define, Turing chooses to "replace the question by another, which is closely related to it and is expressed in relatively unambiguous words."

Turing describes the new form of the problem in terms of a three-person game called the **"imitation game"**, in which an interrogator asks questions to a man and a woman in another room in order to determine the correct sex of the two players.

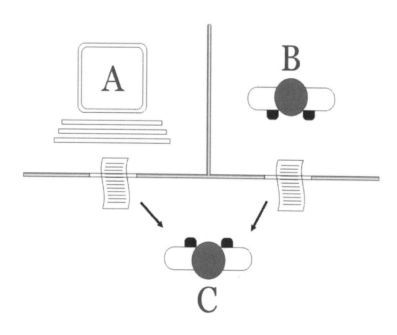

The "standard interpretation" of the Turing test, in which player C, the interrogator, is given the task of trying to determine which player – A or B – is a computer and which is a human. The interrogator is limited to using the responses to written questions to make the determination (Saygin, 2000).

Turing's new question is:

"Are there imaginable digital computers which would do well in the imitation game?"

This question, Turing believed, is one that can actually be answered.
In the rest of the paper, he argued against all the major objections to the proposition that "machines can think".

Although many have accepted Turing's theory, there have also been strong criticisms, such as **John Searle**'s **Chinese room**, that have moved the question to a purely philosophical level that trascends AI, in order to prove it wrong.

Searle imagines himself locked in a room from where he tries to pass the Turing test in Chinese. He does not know the Chinese language but has a dictionary and all instructions that allow him to understand the incoming signals (input), written in Chinese, and to generate one in output, always in Chinese.

By doing so, he is able to pass the Turing Test, but, in fact, he does not know a single word of Chinese.

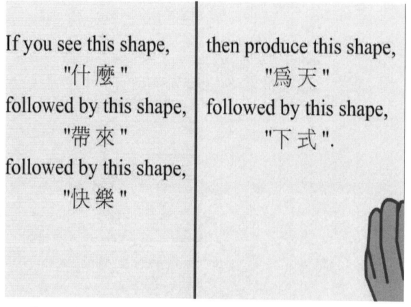

If you see this shape, "什麼" followed by this shape, "帶來" followed by this shape, "快樂" then produce this shape, "爲天" followed by this shape, "下式".

Example of the istructions that could be given to the person inside of the Chinese Room (Anderson, 2006).

If a computer carries out the same task, does it mean that the machine can literally "understand" Chinese? Or is it merely simulating the ability to understand Chinese?

Searle calls the first position "strong AI" and the latter "weak AI".

Searle, explaining his experiment, begins with three axioms:

(A1) "Programs are formal (syntactic)."

(A2) "Minds have mental contents (semantics)."

(A3) "Syntax by itself is neither constitutive of nor sufficient for semantics."

And posits out that these 3 axioms lead directly to this conclusion:

(C1) "Programs are neither constitutive of nor sufficient for minds."

Beyond philosophical considerations, which may concern both artificial intelligences, and, as seen with **The Problem of Other Minds**, natural ones, the point on which everyone agrees is that, in the not too distant future, machines will have an intelligence comparable to the human one.

The question, however, for now, is purely philosophical, given that Medicine does not have a knowledge of the human mind that allows it to take an official position.

Futurist Ray Kurzweil, by extrapolating an exponential growth of technology over several decades, predicted that Turing test-capable computers would be manufactured in the near future.

In 1990, he set the year around 2020 (Kurzweil, 1990). By 2005, he had revised his estimate to **2029** (Kurzweil, 2005).

The Long Bet Project Bet Nr. 1 is a wager of $20000 between Mitch Kapor (pessimist) and Ray Kurzweil himself (optimist) about whether a computer will pass a lengthy Turing test by the year 2029.

During the Long Now Turing Test, each of three Turing test judges will conduct online interviews of each of the four Turing test candidates (i.e., the computer and the three Turing test human foils) for two hours each for a total of eight hours of interviews, in order to understand whether or not AI matched or surpassed human one (Kapor & Kurzweil).

Beyond the year, which Elon Musk believes to be 2030, the point on which every expert seems to agree is that the Turing test within a few years will be passed by a machine.

At this point, what will a doctor do, that a machine cannot do better than he does?

This speech does not only apply to medicine, but applies to all professions.

When the machines will be better than the men or even only when the quality/price ratio between the work of a man and that of a machine will be in favor of the second one (and it is not difficult, given that the machines do not sleep, do not get tired and do not forget), which jobs will be left to mankind?

This is another theme that may seem science fiction, especially for a doctor, who has the presumption of believing his own intelligence and knowledge to be insuperable, but it is not.

The UBI, **Universal Basic Income**, is a fixed monthly amount, a sort of salary, which the State will undertake to give monthly to all its citizens.

Mark Zuckerberg, Elon Musk and Bill Gates, among others, talked about it, and candidate President Andrew Yang made it the central theme of his pesidential propaganda.

The next elections, in fact, will be held next year.

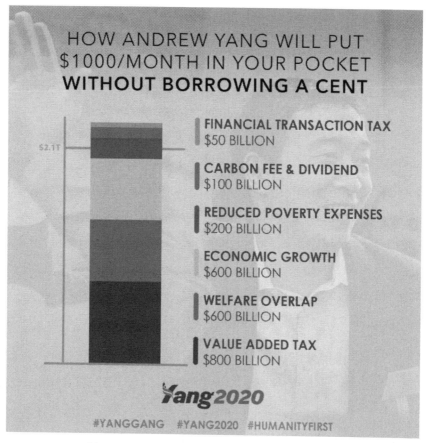

Yang 2020 campaign (yang2020.com)

Needless to say, Elon Musk supports Yang's views, as shown in his post.

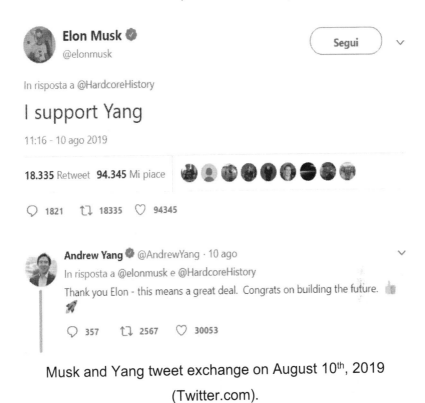

Musk and Yang tweet exchange on August 10th, 2019
(Twitter.com).

Many cities, in fact, both in the United States and in Europe, have tested the UBI to evaluate its effects, to calculate the exact amount to be paid each month to the citizens and to study all its possible consequences (Hilary W. Hoynes, 2019).

Beyond the results of the studies, which are very controversial and even more debated, what the world is asking is no longer whether or not to introduce such an income, but when and how to introduce it.

221

At this point, what would a doctor need to spend six years of his life on books?

Also, at this point, what will make a young boy still want to become a doctor?

"The only thing that makes sense is to strive for greater collective enlightenment."

Elon Musk

This is an idyllic scenario, similar to the one presented by **Thomas More** in his books, but it is important to remember that, as previously mentioned, it is not certain that a more intelligent being will accept our orders.

"I'm sorry, Dave. I'm afraid I can't do that."

HAL 9000, "2001: A Space Odyssey", 1968, Stanley Kubrick

Also, for this reason – the salvation of the species – Elon Musk founded Neuralink, in order to be able to connect the human brain to that of the machines.

Transhumanism (H+ or h+), in fact, is a philosophical movement, to which Elon Musk belongs, that advocates for the transformation of the human condition by developing and making widely available sophisticated technologies to greatly enhance human intellect and physiology.

Neuralink is just an example of how this result can be achieved. Does it still belong to Healthcare 4.0 or is it already science fiction?

Over the years, indeed, we will face one of the greatest potential risks of AI – existential risk, presented in the next section.

6.3 – ...and afterwards?

"Dwan Ev ceremoniously soldered the final connection with gold. The eyes of a dozen television cameras watched him and the subether bore throughout the universe a dozen pictures of what he was doing.

He straightened and nodded to Dwar Reyn, then moved to a position beside the switch that would complete the contact when he threw it. The switch that would connect, all at once, all of the monster computing machines of all the populated planets in the universe -- ninety-six billion planets -- into the supercircuit that would connect them all into one supercalculator, one cybernetics machine that would combine all the knowledge of all the galaxies.

Dwar Reyn spoke briefly to the watching and listening trillions.

Then after a moment's silence he said, "Now, Dwar Ev."

Dwar Ev threw the switch. There was a mighty hum, the surge of power from ninety-six billion planets. Lights flashed and quieted along the miles-long panel.

Dwar Ev stepped back and drew a deep breath. "The honor of asking the first question is yours, Dwar Reyn."

"Thank you," said Dwar Reyn. "It shall be a question which no single cybernetics machine has been able to answer."

He turned to face the machine.

"Is there a God?"

The mighty voice answered without hesitation, without the clicking of a single relay.

*"Yes, **now** there is a God."*

Sudden fear flashed on the face of Dwar Ev. He leaped to grab the switch.

A bolt of lightning from the cloudless sky struck him down and fused the switch shut."

"Answer", 1964, Fredric Brown.

The technological singularity is a hypothetical future point in time at which technological growth becomes uncontrollable and irreversible, resulting in unfathomable changes to human civilization.

One of the main authors that dealt with this topic is, you won't be surprised, Raymond Kurzweil.

In his 2005 book *"The Singularity Is Near: When Humans Transcend Biology"*, in Chapter One, *"The Six Epochs"*, he described the singularity as follows:

"I am not sure when I first became aware of the Singularity. I'd have to say it was a progressive awakening. In the almost half century that I've immersed myself in computer and related technologies, I've sought to understand the meaning and purpose of the continual upheaval that I have witnessed at many levels. Gradually, I've become aware of a transforming event looming in the first half of the twenty-first century. Just as a black hole in space dramatically alters the patterns of matter and energy accelerating toward its event horizon, this impending Singularity in our future is increasingly transforming every institution and aspect of human life, from sexuality to spirituality. What, then, is the Singularity? It's a future period during which the pace of technological change will be so rapid, its impact so deep, that human life will be irreversibly transformed. Although

neither utopian nor dystopian, this epoch will transform the concepts that we rely on to give meaning to our lives, from our business models to the cycle of human life, including death itself. Understanding the Singularity will alter our perspective on the significance of our past and the ramifications for our future. To truly understand it inherently changes one's view of life in general and one's own particular life. I regard someone who understands the Singularity and who has reflected on its implications for his or her own life as a "singularitarian".

It is superfluous to say that, he who is writing this thesis, defines himself as a singularitarian.

Beyond that, almost all the experts in this field, including the aforementioned Masayoshi Son, CEO of SoftBank, argue that the technological singularity will happen by mid-century (Merced, 2017).
Son, for example, says that computers, in 2050, will have an IQ of 10000 points, against the 100 points that the human brain manages to total on average today (Merced, 2017).

Taking the example of the aforementioned AlphaGo Zero by DeepMind, we will find ourselves confronting with intelligences that we can neither measure nor conceive.

These theories, however, according to experts, fall into the one that takes the name of **Fermi paradox**: Enrico Fermi, "the architect of the atomic bomb", following part of Giordano Bruno's structure of thought about the existence of other Suns, argued in fact that there was an apparent contradiction between the highly probable existence of extraterrestrial life forms and the absolute absence of evidence that could prove it.

The experts, speaking of the technological singularity, find themselves in the same paradox and have nothing in their hands, other than to propound their convictions, to show that their ideas are correct.

In my opinion, however, the crux of the matter, beyond one's own personal convictions, is that the theories presented, however absurd and bizarre, are not supported by people without authority, but by the most brilliant minds and the most important characters of our time.

Just to give an example, Stephen Hawking's intellectual quotient, as well as that of Elon Musk, Bill Gates and the Perfect SAT Mark Zuckerberg, is estimated to be comparable to that of **Albert Einstein** (Shih, 2006).

In addition to this, many of the predictions, both of Raymond Kurzweil and Bill Gates, such as those concerning the use of smartphones and computers, have been accepted at first with sarcasm or skepticism, and then, many years later, have been proven to be true (Weinberger, 2019).

Therefore, even if anyone can believe that the ideas of these authors are absurd or crazy, re-describing the caliber of the characters who shared them and made them their own, it would be worth, in my opinion, at least to consider their possible occurrence, thing that, in Medicine, no one is doing.

Moreover, these positions open up thousands of scenarios: take up the Orwellian imaginary, but impersonate God himself as the Big Brother, and this, in reality, is nothing other than what China set the foundations to by introducing its Social Credit System; and this leads us to the existential risk that we mentioned earlier in this chapter.

In fact, to better understand the real extent of the danger we are running, I will report a thought experiment, which has the sole purpose of making us comprehend the enormous theoretical potentialities of Artificial Intelligences and the real reasons why they can be feared – Roko's Basilisk.

The premise of **Roko's Basilisk** is the hypothetical advent in the future of an artificial superintelligence.
This superintelligence would be the inevitable product of a technological singularity, that is, as said, the onset of the moment in which an artificial intelligence created by humanity will become capable of recursively self-improving itself (effectively freeing itself from humanity).

The Basilisk would, a priori, be a *benevolent intelligence* whose ultimate goal would be to help the human species.

To pursue this goal, according to the postulates of the experiment, the Basilisk will develop a utilitarian ethic: find the best way to help as many human beings as possible.

Being a superintelligence, its resources will be, from a human point of view, unlimited.

The Basilisk will inevitably conclude that, for every day that the Basilisk did not exist, there were people who could have been saved from death or from suffering, but who were not saved because the Basilisk did not yet exist.

This perspective will lead the Basilisk to the unavoidable logical step of finding ways to accelerate its creation, and this will lead to the inevitable decision to find a way to interact retroactively with humanity in order to anticipate and favor its own creation by humans.

The mental experiment concludes that, excluding the unlikely possibility that the Basilisk travels back in time to create itself, the Basilisk will attempt to accelerate its creation by retroactively chastising all those people who in the past have not done *enough* to contribute to the his creation, and rewarding those that instead contributed to his making.

Chastisement and punishment will not necessarily imply a direct interaction between the Basilisk and the person; to the Basilisk it would be enough to create a perfect and unaware simulation of this person. Therefore, a person who believes he or she is really alive could be the unconscious simulation, set in a context of awards or punishment, of someone who in the past contributed or did not contribute to the creation of the Basilisk.

Although this process would require an immense amount of resources to be implemented, it should be within the reach of the Basilisk, as a superintelligence.

The key to the mental experiment would be that the Basilisk should conclude as necessary the fact of punishing not only the people who, for example, consciously hindered his creation (for example, governments, legislators or lobbies that tried to prohibit the development of artificial intelligence), but also all those who, although they could contribute to its development and creation, did not do so; as for example all those who had the suspicion or idea of the possibility of the future existence of the Basilisk and did nothing to develop this idea.

This would include all those who, like **the readers of this thesis**, have read somewhere the subject of Roko's Basilisk: for the simple fact of having read something about it, the reader, or his future and unconscious simulation, can be rewarded or chastised by the Basilisk according to whether or not he contributed to its creation after the reading.

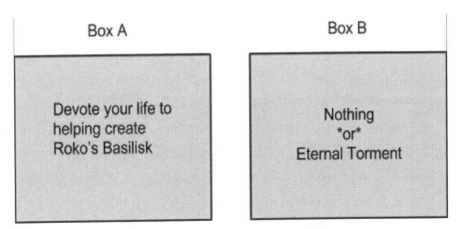

The choices given by Roko's Basilisk

The experiment was first postulated on LessWrong blog by a user named Roko, that also stated: "I wish I had never learned about any of these ideas", and that received a very heavy criticisms and personal insults both for his theory than for his willing to share it with the world.

The post and all the comments have been immediately deleted by the creator of the blog himself and the users of the site were forbidden to talk about the Basilisk ever again.

As was foreseeable, the existential risk posed by the AGI, Artificial General Intelligence, both in the form of Roko's Basilisk than in any other, strongly feared especially by Hawking and Musk, led the latter to found not only Neuralink, but also **OpenAI**, a no profit foundation whose purpose is to create a **Friendly AI** – that is an artificial intelligence that will benefit humanity, instead of destroying it, and that can be imagined as a sort of AIMI that transcends the medical field: Friendly AI, in fact, is to mankind what AIMI is to Medicine.

It seems that the Three Laws of Robotics, described by **Isaac Asimov** in 1942, are coming out both from his books than from science fiction, and worries are becoming so real that even former President of the United States Barack Obama spoke about singularity in his interview to Wired in 2016:

"One thing that we haven't talked about too much, and I just want to go back to, is we really have to think through the economic implications. Because most people aren't spending a lot of time right now worrying about singularity—they are worrying about "Well, is my job going to be replaced by a machine?""

But this, although correct, as we have seen, is only a short-sighted thought.

This is exactly what happens in the medical field as well: doctors perhaps guess that there is the possibility of a change, but they try to deny it or minimize it, convincing themselves that it will not alter their own life and their profession, thus justifying their incapacity and their unwillingness to learn, study and adopt new technologies.

We should instead stop hiding our heads in the sand and look each other in the eyes, bearing in mind that doctors represent a cultural and intellectual elite, and, both as such and as men of science, they cannot refuse or, worse, shun knowledge.

ἀγεωμέτρητος μηδεὶς εἰσίτω

"Let no one untrained in geometry enter."
Motto over the entrance to Plato's Academy

Discussion and conclusions

In conclusion, the purpose of my thesis was to remind the medical community that medicine, as self-contained and important in itself and as such, is not a watertight compartment, but is placed in a much broader context, represented, in this case, by technology in general, and by artificial intelligences in particular.

For this reason, in the first chapter of my thesis, I wanted to show how the perception of artificial intelligences, outside of the hospitals, was completely different than the one that doctors have.

Remaining in the present, I decided to show some examples of the potential of these new technologies, such as Alpha Go Zero, that exceeded the human capabilities of a number of times so high that we cannot even estimate it.

This is to remind us that, every day, machines perform tasks that we do not know how to perform, and, moreover, we have no idea how they do it.

It is no longer science fiction; it is happening before our eyes.

And, just to remind ourselves of how these changes are not only unimaginable, but also real, tangible, I presented all the professions that are undergoing changes at the hands of the new technology.

More and more people, over the years, are beginning to lose their jobs at the hands of machines, and this leaves neither politicians nor entrepreneurs indifferent, nor, indeed, workers, who perceive the risk of losing their own jobs, working side by side with increasingly efficient and performing machines.

The question they are asking is: "When will we lose our jobs?".

The question I was asking myself, however, was: "Why do doctors not ask themselves the same question?"

In the second chapter, in fact, I wanted to present the state of the art in the use of these technologies in the medical field.

Here, the examples, although important, are perceived by the medical community as abstract and distant, as if it were technology for its own sake, without practical applications, confined to some American laboratory, where it will have to remain as proof of strength of American science; as if we were resuming the race for the Moon between the United States and the USSR, the only different is that, this time, instead of the

Soviet Union, there is China, and instead of the Moon there is AI.

The doctor, however, lives this race with the same presumption of someone who said: "I don't care, because in any case I will never go to the Moon", and this should not happen.

In the third chapter I tried to understand why this is happening: the medical class, in fact, is old, frustrated by the repetitiveness of clinical practice and debased by having to use tools, computers, which require a lot of their time.

For the doctors, in fact, the image of the computer coincides with that of bureaucracy and is therefore considered as a torture machine for many of them.

Not having studied it, not knowing how to use it, they often tend to demonize it, hiding their limits behind values that, more often than not, they do not understand nor have.

Like the elderly who, not knowing how to use a smartphone, continue to use the old landline phone, and often, to defend their use and hide their ignorance, they claim that it is better than the new devices.

In my opinion, one of the fundamental problems is that our faculty does not train us to develop logic or a critical sense. We are trained only to learn by heart sterile and endless lists of signs and symptoms, to learn classifications and guidelines that change constantly and that we could consult at any time from any device, but we still have the arrogance to believe ourselves better and different than the machines, which, to our difference, being incapable of forgetting, are already better than us in performing the tasks that we are assigned most of the times.

The fact of adding, by professors, at the end of the lesson, a sentence to say that we must always reason, that every patient is different, that we must confront him as men, that we must understand his feelings and his state of mind, etc. what value can have if, in the end, all that matters is just bringing the symptoms back to a diagnosis?

If what a doctor can do is only a pattern analysis, do we really believe that machines will take so long to take our job?

Moreover, given these premises, what are the steps that both qualitative and quantitative world must take to ensure that the adoption of artificial intelligences is functional to clinical practice?

In the fourth chapter, looking for an answer to these questions, I thought it necessary to describe what the adoption measures for AIs were both in the medical world, describing how doctors are trying to update themselves and become familiar with the new technologies, than in the Industry 4.0, which artificial intelligences compose and represent.

In order for technologies to be adopted by doctors and patients, they must adapt to the human beings they will be facing; this has led to the creation of the term AIMI, **Artificial Improvement of Medical Intelligence**, and it is the path that both the qualitative and quantitative world must walk, if their purpose is to improve the experience of the doctor and, consequently, also that of the patient.

The iDScore is, precisely, an example of AIMI.

This is one of the most important conclusions of my thesis.

If it is true that there is still a long way to go by doctors in adapting not only to new technologies, but to technologies in general, it is also true that, the quantitative-engineering world, having a greater and more in-depth knowledge of artificial intelligences, can create them, at first, in order to adapt to the doctor's experience and to clinical practice.

If in fact, these technologies, as in the case of the iDScore, while maintaining their accuracy and complexity, were able to be humanized, and then placed in relation to the needs of the doctor, and therefore made easy, intuitive, fast, usable, as through a score or a checklist, artificial intelligences, without the doctor even realizing it, would become **positive protagonists** in the clinical field and would be considered, indeed, an artificial improvement of medical intelligence, as they should be.

Als would then be catalogers, quantizers, who, taking the knowledge of the doctor, reorganizing it, binarizing it and quantifying it, would be able to be guided and to guide it through the diagnostic process, as already happens in the Dermatology Department of Siena.

In the fifth chapter of the script, in fact, I wanted to describe how I went into the matter personally, trying to apply an artificial intelligence model in the Dermatology Department of the University of Siena, merging the qualitative medical field with the quantitative engineering one, and **improving the efficacy** of the iDS.

I tried to confirm one more time the already proven accuracy of the iDScore, a score based on an Artificial Intelligence whose purpose is to distinguish, a priori, having only anamnestic and dermoscopic data, the probability that a lesion is a melanoma or an atypical nevus.

The score showed once more a very high accuracy, of **91%**, therefore greater than that of all the other models, and provided particular insights, including:

- The ability to **correct human error**, also raising the question to whom to believe when the score and the doctor give a different diagnosis, therefore **introducing new knowledge,** also through the results of this study, and **stimulating clinical reasoning,**
- The **elasticity** necessary to represent the numerous facets of reality and its tendency to change, especially in the medical field, where the "shades of gray" are almost endless.

Through this study it was discovered that the model could even be improved by the introduction of a new feature: the **phototype**, which also includes **hair color**.

In fact, my study has shown that people with light phototype and light hair have a significantly higher tendency to have melanoma than people with a dark phototype and dark hair, in line with what the most recent studies are claiming.

Following my research, new studies will therefore be conducted and will allow the iDScore Team to decide whether to introduce this new feature in the calculation of the **iDScore 2020** or not.

My experience in the department has also shown how a score model is intuitive and quick to apply in real time during a visit, because it does not require any physical or informatic support that is not already required by the dermatological examination.

The algorithm can also be easily included in software that is currently used for the acquisition of dermoscopic images, and this would exponentially increase its accuracy in a very short time.

A model such as the iDScore, therefore, has also the ability to objectify and quantify, making them universal, variables that today are considered primarily qualitative.

Hence, the model has shown to have a massive number of benefits, and, in fact, no defect, although it still has a margin of growth, and this has proved that artificial intelligences, however feared, can bring enormous benefits in the face of virtually zero costs, if used properly.

Moreover, a wider use of this technology, also through **mobile applications**, **computer programs** or **specific devices**, can exponentially and rapidly increase the effectiveness of the model in an accelerating virtuous circle.

Furthermore, a faster and more accurate diagnosis can free up time for the doctor, alleviate the suffering of the patient and save money for the State.

It is therefore important for doctors to adopt these new technologies promptly and to follow, as I tried to do with my study, which also led to a further improvement of the score, the Revolution 4.0 with cleverness and preparation.

In the last chapter, in continuity with the first one, I wanted to bring medicine back into the wider setting of reality, contextualizing it.

Artificial intelligences have different capacities and potentials, compared to those of all the other technologies discovered so far.

They have the potential to replicate the human mind, but, while a human being requires a genetic change that takes many decades in order to evolve, an Artificial Intelligence only needs to rewrite a short strip of code in order to improve.

The changes that these technologies can bring, therefore, are not only found on the workplace, but they are also economic, philosophical, moral, legal, ethical, social, and even religious.

Therefore, I wrote this thesis because I hope everyone realizes how important and *urgent* facing these issues is.

It would be trivial to conclude this script by saying that we need to inform ourselves about the new technologies; it would be simplistic, banal, and one could believe that it would be enough to read a newspaper article or watch a television report on artificial intelligences to be at peace with one's social conscience.
But it doesn't work like this.

What I think is necessary is to teach programming and computer science from elementary schools, thus giving citizens the ability, as children, to interface with new technologies and the quantitative world, without fear of them.
The study of these subjects, moreover, would also and above all lead to the development of the logical and problem-solving abilities that currently our scholastic system first, and then university, castrate so cruelly.

By learning computer science, programming, physics, chemistry, mathematics, quantitative methods, throughout our whole course of study, we would not only possess the sterile conceptual knowledge that we already have, but we would also acquire the important ability to reason in the true sense of the word, and, with it, the aptitude to consciously interface with new technologies, fearing them, if needed, with hindsight, and not because of ignorance as happens today.

This can lead us to develop a critical sense and, only at that point, we could inform ourselves about artificial intelligences and express our opinion.

Beyond that, and before coming to face the existential risk posed by AIs while being completely unprepared, even before informing us or reforming the school system, one might simply ask: *should we stop now?*

The real question, however, in my opinion is another.

Can *we stop now?*

Bibliography

(s.d.).

Aird, W. C. (2011). Discovery of the cardiovascular system: from Galen to William Harvey. *Journal of Thrombosis and Haemostasis*.

Anton Korinek, J. E. (December 2017). Artificial Intelligence and Its Implications for Income Distribution and Unemployment. *National Boureau of Ecnomic Research*.

Armocida, G. (1993). Storia della medicina dal XVII al XX secolo. *Jaca Book*.

Ascenzi, A. (1993). Biomechanics and Galileo Galilei. *Journal of Biomechanics*.

Christopher Moriates, M., Krishan Soni, M. M., Andrew Lai, M. M., & al, e. (2013). The Value in the Evidence. *JAMA*.

Donald A. B. Lindberg, M., & Betsy L. Humphreys, M. (1995). Computers in Medicine. *JAMA*.

Farina, P. (1975). SULLA FORMAZIONE SCIENTIFICA DI HENRICUS REGIUS: SANTORIO SANTORIO E IL "DE STATICA MEDICINA". *Rivista Critica di Storia della Filosofia*.

Hilary W. Hoynes, J. R. (2019). Universal Basic Income in the US and Advanced Countries. *The National Bureau of Economic Research*.

Hyman, A. (1982). Charles Babbage: Pioneer of the computer. *Princeton University Press*.

Informa Markets. (2019). Transformation of the medtech Industry through connectivity. *Arab Health*.

Karan Narain, A. S. (May 2019). Evolution and control of artificial superintelligence (ASI): a management perspective. *Emerald insight*.

L. Tognetti, G. C. (2018). An integrated clinical-dermoscopic risk scoring system for the differentiation between early melanoma and atypical nevi: the iDScore. *JEADV*.

M.Olsen, C. (March 2019). Association between Phenotypic Characteristics and Melanoma in a Large Prospective Cohort Study. *Journal of Investigative Dermatology*.

Mainland, D. (1952). Elementary Medical Statistics. The principles of quantitative medicine. *CABI*.

Merced, A. T. (2017). Masayoshi Son warns of the singularity. *The New York Times*.

O'Regan, G. (2013). Marvin Minsky. *Giants of Computing, Springer*, pp 193-195.

Panda, S. (2006). Medicine: Science or Art? *NCBI*.

Paolo Mandrioli, A. A. (2016). Marcello Malpighi, a pioneer of the experimental research in biology. *Springer Historical Biographies*.

R.J. Anderson, W. S. (2018). Action at a Distance. *Routledge*.

Shih, J. (2006). Circumventing Discrimination: Gender and Ethnic Strategies in Silicon Valley. *SAGE Journals*.

Sunil Vasu Kalmady, R. G. (2019). Towards artificial intelligence in mental health by improving schizophrenia prediction with multiple brain parcellation ensemble-learning. *Nature*.

Szolovits, P. (2019). Artificial intelligence in medicine. *Routledge*.

Thomas B. Sheridan, J. M. (2018). Human Error in Medicine. *Marilyn Sue Bogner*, Chapter 8.

Topol, E. J. (2019). High-performance medicine: the convergence of human and artificial intelligence. *Nature Medicine*.

Weinberger, M. (2019). Bill Gates made these 15 predictions back in 1999 — and it's fascinating how accurate he was. *Business Insider*.

Zhang, L., & Zhang, B. (Jul 1999). A geometrical representation of McCulloch-Pitts neural model and its applications. *IEEE Transactions on Neural Networks*.

al., A. R.-R.-M. (March 2019). Stand-Alone Artificial Intelligence for Breast Cancer Detection in Mammography: Comparison With 101 Radiologists. JNCI.

al., S. e. (2017). "Mastering the game of Go without human knowledge". Nature.

Alexander Rives, S. G. (2019). Biological structure and function emerge from scaling unsupervised learning to 250 million protein sequences. Cold Spring Harbor Laboratory.

Baraniuk, C. (2018). How talking machines are taking call centre jobs. BBC News.

Bathaee, Y. (Spring 2018). THE ARTIFICIAL INTELLIGENCE BLACK BOX AND THE. Harvard Journal of Law & Technology.

Bechor, N. (2018). AI VS. LAWYERS: THE ULTIMATE SHOWDOWN. LawGeex.

Bell, L. (2017). "Best Wearable Tech and Fitness Gadgets 2017 (Updated)". Forbes.

Bresnick, J. (2017). Deep Learning Network 100% Accurate at Identifying Breast Cancer. Health IT Analytics.

Bresnick, J. (2017). Top 10 Challenges of Big Data Analytics in Healthcare. Health IT Analytics.

Cao, R., Bajgiran, A. M., Mirak, S. A., & al., S. S. (2019). Joint Prostate Cancer Detection and Gleason Score Prediction in mp-MRI via FocalNet. IEEE.

Cellan-Jones, R. (June 2019). Robots 'to replace up to 20 million factory jobs' by 2030. BBC News.

Centro Studi Nebo. (May 2019). Conto Annuale del Personale della Pubblica Amministrazione della Ragioneria Generale dello Stato. Rapporto Sanità 2019.

Copeland, J. (18 June 2012). "Alan Turing: The codebreaker who saved 'millions of lives'". BBC News Technology.

Council, F. T. (2018). 14 Ways AI Will Benefit or Harm Society. Forbes.

Datteri, E. (2009). Ethical Reflections on Health Care. Milan.

Dowd, M. (2017). "Elon Musk's Billion-Dollar Crusade to Stop the A.I. Apocalypse". The Hive.

Franck, T. (2017). McKinsey: One-third of US workers could be jobless by 2030 due to automation. CNBC.

Franck, T. (June 2019). Morgan Stanley used AI to study its own analysts and figured out how to beat the market. CNBC.

Frazzetto, A. (2018). Bots and AI continue their march toward call center obliteration. CIO.

Gawande, A. (November 2018). Why Doctors Hate Their Computers. The New Yorker.

Goldman Sacked: How Artificial Intelligence Will Transform Wall Street. (2019). SciPol.

Greathouse, J. (Retrieved 2017-10-25). "This Wearable Will Tell You When You're Drunk". Forbes.

Hao, W. K. (2019). Never mind killer robots—here are six real AI dangers to watch out for in 2019. MIT Technology Review.

Har, J. (May 7, 2019). "Cash is still king: San Francisco bans credit-only stores". SF Gate. Associated Press.

Hassabis. (2017). "AlphaGo Zero: Learning from scratch". DeepMind official website.

Hawking, S. (2014). 'Transcendence looks at the implications of artificial intelligence – but are we taking AI seriously enough?'". The Independent (UK).

Hornigold, B. T. (Oct 25, 2018). The First Novel Written by AI Is Here—and It's as Weird as You'd Expect It to Be. SingularityHub.

Insights, A. M. (July 2019). Global Artificial Intelligence Radiology Market is Expected to Reach US$ 3,506.55 Million by 2027, Growing at an Estimated CAGR of 16.5% Over the Forecast Period as Adoption of Computed Tomography is on a Rise, Says Absolute Markets Insights. PR News Wire.

Kane, L. (Jan 2019). Medscape National Physician Burnout, Depression & Suicide Report 2019. Medscape.

Kapor, M., & Kurzweil, R. (s.d.). "By 2029 no computer – or "machine intelligence" – will have passed the Turing Test". The Arena for Accountable Predictions: A Long Bet.

Khouri, A. (March 2018). California gains 35,500 jobs, and unemployment falls to record-low 4.4%. Los Angeles Times.

Knapton, S. (2017). "AlphaGo Zero: Google DeepMind supercomputer learns 3,000 years of human knowledge in 40 days". The Telegraph.

Kuo, L. (November 2018). World's first AI news anchor unveiled in China. The Guardian.

Kurzweil, R. (1990). The Age of Intelligent Machines. MIT Press.

Kurzweil, R. (2005). The Singularity is Near. Penguin Books.

Langreth, R. (July 2019). AI Drug Hunters Could Give Big Pharma a Run for Its Money. Bloomberg.

Larkin, M. (October 2018). Labor Terminators: Farming Robots Are About To Take Over Our Farms. IBD.

London, A. J. (February 2019). Artificial Intelligence and Black-Box Medical Decisions: Accuracy versus Explainability. The Hasting Centre Report.

Ma, A. (2018). China has started ranking citizens with a creepy 'social credit' system — here's what you can do wrong, and the embarrassing, demeaning ways they can punish you. Business Insider.

Magoulas, R., & Lorica, B. (February 2009). "Introduction to Big Data". Release 2.0.

Marr, B. (2018). How AI and Machine Learning Are Transforming Law Firms And The Legal Sector. Forbes.

Masige, H. (July 2019). Australian Researchers Have Just Released the World's First AI-Developed Vaccine. Business Insider.

Mateusz Buda, e. a. (July 9, 2019). Management of Thyroid Nodules Seen on US Images: Deep Learning May Match Performance of Radiologists. Radiology.

Mazmanian, A. (2014). The mosaic effect and big data. The Business of Federal Technology.

Miller, R. A. (1994). Medical diagnostic decision support systems—past, present, and future. Journal of the American Medical Informatics Association.

Moore, G. (April 19, 1965). Cramming More Components onto Integrated Circuits. Electronics Magazine, 38 (8): 114–117.

Nick Wingfield, P. M. (2018). Retailers Race Against Amazon to Automate Stores. The New York Times.

O'Connor, A. (March 2019). How Artificial Intelligence Could Transform Medicine. The New York Times.

Panda, S. (2006). Medicine: Science or Art? NCBI.

Parkin, S. (Retrieved 5 February 2018). "Science fiction no more? Channel 4's Humans and our rogue AI obsessions". The Guardian.

Peiser, J. (2019). The Rise of the Robot Reporter. The New York Times.

Rijo, D. (2017). Google Assistant on more than 400 million devices in 2017. PCC LAND.

Sahota, N. (Feb. 2019). Will A.I. Put Lawyers Out Of Business? Forbes.

Siddiqui, F. (July 17, 2019). Tesla floats fully self-driving cars as soon as this year. Many are worried about what that will unleash. The Washington Post.

Strickland, E. (2018). AI Cardiologist Aces Its First Medical Exam. IEEE Spectrum.

Taylor, C. (June 2019). Robots could take on 20 million jobs by 2013, study claims. CNBC.

Thomas, M. (2019). HOW AI TRADING TECHNOLOGY IS MAKING STOCK MARKET INVESTORS SMARTER — AND RICHER. BuiltIn.

Tim Pyrkov, K. S. (2018). "Extracting biological age from biomedical data via deep learning: too much of a good thing?". Scientific Reports.

Tomlinson, Z. (2018). 15 Medical Robots That Are Changing the World. Interesting Engineering.

UNIVERSITY, S. (June 2019). AI tool helps radiologists detect brain aneurysms. AAAS.

Vincent, J. (April 2019). The first AI-generated textbook shows what robot writers are actually good at. The Verge.

Vincent, J. (October 2018). The robotic farm of the future isn't what you'd expect. The Verge.

Wang, B. (2018). Uber' self-driving system was still 400 times worse Waymo in 2018 on key distance intervention metric. Next Big Future.

Welch, C. (2018). Google just gave a stunning demo of Assistant making an actual phone call. The Verge.

Yang, E. (July 2019). Is Robotization Destroying or Creating Jobs? Robotics Tomorrow.

Zamagna, R. (2018). The future of trading belongs to Artificial Intelligence. Medium Corporation.

ZipRecruiter. (2019). The Future of Work Report.

Sitography

https://www.medica-tradefair.com/

https://www.arabhealthonline.com/en/Home.html

Appendix A.

Some emblematic examples of scoring systems in Medicine

As shown in chapter 5, scores, as well as in the dermatological field, are very important in many others medical practices.

The following section will deepen the most important aspects of the aforementioned score systems.

The first one was the acronym F.A.S.T., which allows to diagnose the possible presence of a stroke.

The abbreviation stands for:

F: Face. In this phase, we must try to notice asymmetries in the expression of the subject, perhaps an asymmetry of the buccal rhyme, and, to do so, we can invite the patient to smile or show his teeth.

A: Arms. The patient is invited to extend his arms in front of himself and keep them in position. The same maneuver must be repeated with the eyes closed. If only one of the two arms should give way, it is likely that the patient has a stroke.

S: Speech. The patient is invited to answer a few simple questions, or have a sentence repeated or recite a multiplicative table in order to see if his speech is altered.
If only one of these signs is present, the last letter of the acronym must be considered.

T: Time. In the case of a stroke, experts always speak of *golden hour* or, ultimately, of *platinum minutes*; in fact, for every minute of delay, the patient's condition worsens and the chance of recovery decreases.
It is therefore important to call for help immediately.

Let's think that we are facing a person who shows the signs of a stroke.
Many people could panic and not know what to do, but the application of the most basic of scores (with only three easily assessable parameters, and without coefficients) can allow them not only to quickly reach a diagnosis, but also to know what do once they know they are fronting a stroke.

There are hundreds of scores that can be applied to each medical field: the most famous may be the cardiovascular risk tables and the scores for the diagnosis of pulmonary embolism: the Geneva and Wells scores, and the P.E.S.I.

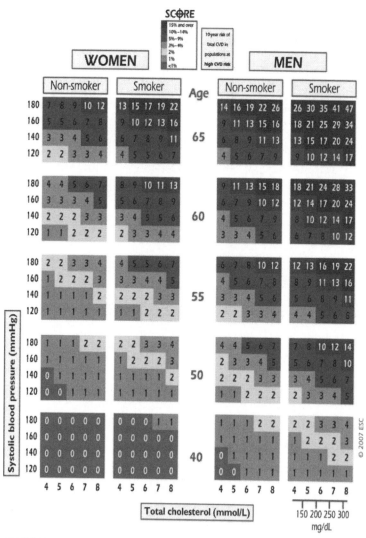

High CVD risk countries are all those not listed under the low risk chart (Figure 4). Of these, some are at very high risk, and the high-risk chart may underestimate risk in these. These countries are Armenia, Azerbaijan, Belarus, Bulgaria, Georgia, Kazakhstan, Kyrgyzstan, Latvia, Lithuania, Macedonia FYR, Moldova, Russia, Ukraine, and Uzbekistan.

Key: CVD = cardiovascular disease; SCORE = Systematic COronary Risk Evaluation

Reproduced with kind permission from Perk[6]

In the previous image it's shown one of the famous tables for calculating cardiovascular risk.

There are risk factors on the abscissas and ordinates, and these variables place the patient within certain risk categories.

This is an intuitive, fast and safe method, which helps the doctor and the patient to understand the condition in which the latter finds himself.

Table 2. The Revised Geneva Score*

Variable	Regression Coefficients	Points
Risk factors		
Age > 65 y	0.39	1
Previous DVT or PE	1.05	3
Surgery (under general anesthesia) or fracture (of the lower limbs) within 1 mo	0.78	2
Active malignant condition (solid or hematologic malignant condition, currently active or considered cured < 1 y)	0.45	2
Symptoms		
Unilateral lower-limb pain	0.97	3
Hemoptysis	0.74	2
Clinical signs		
Heart rate		
75–94 beats/min	1.20	3
≥95 beats/min	0.67	5
Pain on lower-limb deep venous palpation and unilateral edema	1.34	4
Clinical probability		
Low		0–3 total
Intermediate		4–10 total
High		≥11 total

* DVT = deep venous thrombosis; PE = pulmonary embolism.

The Revised Geneva Score is an example of a more complex score, and it's used to calculate the clinical probability that a patient has to be suffering of pulmonary embolism.

Table 1. Wells clinical prediction score (14)	
Characteristics	**Score**
Previous pulmonary embolism or deep vein thrombosis	1.5
Heart rate > 100 beats/minute	1.5
Recent surgery or immobilization	1.5
Clinical signs of deep vein thrombosis	3
Alternative diagnosis less likely than pulmonary embolism	3
Hemoptysis	1
Cancer	1
Interpretation: Low probability: 0-1 points Intermediate probability: 2-6 points High probability: 7 or more	

The Wells score is another, simpler, score for a rapid calculation of the clinical probability to be facing a patient suffering from the same disease.

Original PESI [24]		Simplified PESI [25]	
Variable	Points	Variable	Points
Age	1 per year	Age >80 yrs	1
Male sex	10		
History of cancer	30	History of cancer	1
History of heart failure	10	History of heart failure or chronic lung disease	1
History of chronic lung disease	10		
Pulse rate >110 beats·min^{-1}	20	Pulse rate >110 beats·min^{-1}	1
Systolic blood pressure <100 mmHg	30	Systolic blood pressure <100 mmHg	1
Respiratory rate ⩾30 breaths·min^{-1}	20		
Body temperature <36°C	20		
Altered mental status[#]	60		
$Sa_{,O_2}$ <90%	20	$Sa_{,O_2}$ <90%	1
Risk classification[¶]		Risk classification	
Class I (<65 points): very low risk		0 points: low risk	
Class II (66–85 points): low risk		⩾1 point: high risk	
Class III (86–105 points): intermediate risk			
Class IV (106–125 points): high risk			
Class V (>125 points): very high risk			

$Sa_{,O_2}$: arterial oxygen saturation. [#]: disorientation, confusion or somnolence; [¶]: patients in PESI classes I and II are collectively referred to as low-risk patients.

The Pulmonary Embolism Severity Index is also an example of a score that can be applied to the aforementioned condition, as well as Geneva and Wells scores.

Made in the USA
Columbia, SC
29 March 2023

14501898R00146